# The University of Michigan School of Dentistry

Victors for Dentistry
(1962–2017)

# The University of Michigan School of Dentistry

Victors for Dentistry
(1962–2017)

*Decades of Innovation and Discovery*

SHARON K. GRAYDEN, EDITOR

Published in the United States of America by
Michigan Publishing
Manufactured in the United States of America

DOI: 10.3998/mpub.9973100

ISBN 978-1-60785-458-6 (hardcover)
ISBN 978-1-60785-459-3 (paper)
ISBN 978-1-60785-460-9 (e-book)


An imprint of Michigan Publishing, Maize Books serves the publishing needs of the University of Michigan community by making high-quality scholarship widely available in print and online. It represents a new model for authors seeking to share their work within and beyond the academy, offering streamlined selection, production, and distribution processes. Maize Books is intended as a complement to more formal modes of publication in a wide range of disciplinary areas.

http://www.maizebooks.org

*To all Victors for Dentistry—faculty, staff, students, alumni, and friends—for your unfailing commitment to excellence.*

# Contents

# Foreword

*Victors for Dentistry (1962–2017)* offers a wonderful collection of historical facts that are a significant part of my life as a dental professional. Construction of the "new" School of Dentistry began in 1966, the year that my classmates and I graduated. The progress in moving this school forward since that time has been phenomenal. The dedication of faculty and staff to educate and graduate future leaders in dentistry throughout the years has been steadfast. I have observed with great pride the many accolades and tributes bestowed on this great school.

Professionalism, integrity, compassion, and lifelong learning were four important principles that were instilled in me during my four years in dental school, and I took ownership of these principles after I graduated in 1966. They guided me when I was assigned to the Philippine Islands as an officer in the United States Air Force, where I established myself in clinical practice and forensic dentistry. They guided me when I joined Mott Children's Health Center in Flint, Michigan, to practice pediatric dentistry, and they have been an integral part of the value system that I adhered to as a leader in organized dentistry. It fills me with pride to be a dental school alumnus.

As I perused this rich history of my dental school from 1962 through 2017, I was pleased to see that the administration, faculty, and staff have been, and continue to be, proactive on all fronts. That throughout the decades, administrations have kept the focus on excellence and have worked diligently to ensure a welcoming and effective environment for educating future dental professionals, providing exceptional patient care, and conducting world-class research. The school has clearly developed an ideal formula for maintaining its status as the number one dental school in America.

Also illustrated are the challenges of keeping pace with, and effecting, continual change in dentistry. The School of Dentistry has long recognized the importance of obtaining a balance in the diversification of its student body when reviewing the large number of highly qualified students who apply. The school has made the search for more efficient and effective diagnostic and treatment regimens to provide a quality service for patients a priority. The school's faculty leaders have understood that updates to the strategic plan, including the curriculum, were necessary. They also understood that advances in technology would be a driving force in dental education, patient care, and research.

As you read these pages, you will see that Michigan's faculty members were key thought-leaders in dental education. They could envision the future and were able to apply a unique blend of ingenuity, experience, and creativity in selecting students most likely to succeed, nurturing their talents, and graduating them as outstanding health-care professionals and potential leaders.

I have witnessed the progress and transformation of my dental school throughout this entire period, and I continue to marvel at the vision, dedication, and determination that have been required to maintain its primary position in leadership.

The curriculum was challenging and demanding, but throughout my years in dental school, I was "aggressively encouraged" by my educators to keep moving forward and to stay creative and focused as I completed my clinical and study obligations. The skill set I acquired helped me become an excellent clinician and laid the foundation for the leadership opportunities that followed, culminating in my election to the presidency of the American Dental Association in 2009.

As highlighted in this book, my School of Dentistry is focused on providing the best environment to admit, educate, and graduate leaders in the dental profession, and with all things considered, it takes pride in the knowledge that its graduates are well prepared to pursue their chosen paths with confidence.

It is an immense source of pride for me to know that I am a graduate of the dental school that insists on excellence. No matter where in the world I travel, it is acknowledged that the University of Michigan School of Dentistry commands respect and is recognized for its innovation and the quality of the education it offers.

I hope you enjoy *Victors for Dentistry (1962–2017)*, reflecting on the impressive path our school has taken over the last 55 years, as much as I have. The written history of the University of Michigan School of Dentistry is rich and defining, and as I review the decades of transformation with pleasure, I look to the future as this excellence in leadership continues.

Raymond Gist, DDS 1966
*2009 President, American Dental Association*

# Preface

One of the first things I did when I became Director of Communications in 2008 was to page through the School of Dentistry's *Alumni Bulletin-Centennial Issue 1875–1975*, published as a historical retrospective by Dr. Charles C. Kelsey (DDS 1964, MS 1967), the school's historian at the time. While not a chronology, the Kelsey volume highlights many noteworthy occasions—people involved, images captured, and accomplishments recorded—from when the School of Dentistry was established in 1875 to just before the centennial year. The content has been a wonderful resource for me over the years and the little blue book has occupied a special place on my desk, always within easy reach.

The idea for a follow-up to the Kelsey centennial issue coincided with planning for the 2017 University of Michigan (U-M) Bicentennial celebration. During the summer of 2012, all schools and colleges were asked by the Bicentennial Planning Committee to update their discipline-specific section of the previously published historical record, *The University of Michigan: An Encyclopedic Survey* (Bunting, Russell L. (1945) and Kelsey, Charles C.(1975)). This updated historical summary was to be included in the bicentennial's *University History Initiative (The University of Michigan, An Encyclopedic Survey: Bicentennial Edition)* and become part of the Bentley Historical Library collection. Our submission was to cover the time frame from the 1970s through 2012, and we were limited to a mere 30 pages.

When Dean Laurie McCauley saw the 30-page encyclopedic summary, her immediate response was, "Let's use this as the framework to update our School of Dentistry history." And so began the work to transform the 30-page encyclopedic rendering into a contemporary recap of the life and times of U-M School of Dentistry from the early 1960s to the present day.

*Victors for Dentistry (1962–2017)* is constructed around the eras of leadership from 1962 through 2017. While each dean has left an indelible mark on the school, this book is not a book about the deans. Their guidance and direction has provided a backdrop to showcase some of the phenomenal accomplishments of the faculty, staff, and students in each era. This book is a record of the significant initiatives and achievements that validated Michigan dentistry's commitment to its mission—leading in teaching, research, service, and patient care.

If the first 100 years were years of evolution in dental education, the decades that followed have been nothing short of transformational. The U-M School of Dentistry has always set a high bar, not afraid to challenge the status quo and not content with the way things have always been done. Always asking, "how can we do this better." The narrative starts in 1962 with a proposal for a new dental building and concludes, more than 55 years later, with a proposal for a major building renovation. What lies between is a story of vision and possibility for dental education that is unparalleled anywhere.

This book celebrates all that the professional community known as the U-M School of Dentistry has accomplished. Through good times and times of change, it has always been about the people—the drivers, the visionaries, and the innovators—who persisted regardless of the usual obstacles and inertia that often stand in the path of progress in higher education. They elevated the school to a world-class prominence that most definitely exemplifies the university's history as home to the "leaders and best."

Sharon K. Grayden, Editor
*Director of Communications, 2008–2016*

# Introduction

"This was an era of mega changes."

"We didn't stand still. We were building the future."

Those remarks, the first from former University of Michigan (U-M) School of Dentistry Dean Dr. William Kotowicz and the other from Professor Wendy Kerschbaum, who directed the school's dental hygiene program for 24 years, best summarize what occurred at the School of Dentistry during a span of more than 50 years from the early 1960s through 2017.

During those five plus decades, six men led the School of Dentistry. On September 1, 2013, Dr. Laurie McCauley became the first woman to be named dean of the School of Dentistry. Her appointment was announced in March 2013 by then U-M Provost Dr. Philip Hanlon and approved by Regents.

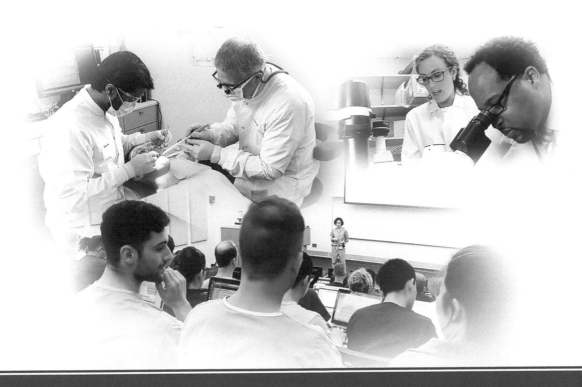

**ADVANCING HEALTH THROUGH EDUCATION, SERVICE, RESEARCH AND DISCOVERY.**

The deans of the U-M School of Dentistry from 1962 to 2017 make up an impressive group of leaders in dental education:

- Dr. William R. Mann (Dean, 1962–1981)

- Dr. Robert E. Doerr (Interim Dean, 1981–1982)

- Dr. Richard L. Christiansen (Dean, 1982–1987)

- Dr. William R. Kotowicz (Interim Dean, 1987–1989)

- Dr. J. Bernard Machen (Dean, 1989–1995)

- Dr. William R. Kotowicz (Acting Dean, 1995–1996; Dean, 1996–2003)

- Dr. Peter J. Polverini (Dean, 2003–2013)

- Dr. Laurie McCauley (Dean, 2013–)

(See Appendix A for a list of all of the people who have held the title of dean of the U-M School of Dentistry.)

This book chronicles more than five decades of innovation and discovery that have distinguished the School of Dentistry and its faculty, staff, and graduates as the leaders and best in dentistry. From the early 1960s through 2017, major changes occurred throughout the School of Dentistry affecting both the physical structure and its programs.

*Victors for Dentistry (1962–2017)* is constructed around eras of leadership, starting with Dean William Mann in 1962 and ending with Dean Laurie McCauley in 2017. Each dean provided a solid foundation upon which faculty, staff, and students could thrive and succeed. Hallmarks of this time period, 1962–2017, include transformational changes to dental and dental hygiene curricula, new approaches to patient care, notable changes in student enrollment, advances in science and technology that translated research findings into clinical practice, and major improvements to facilities. Visionary leaders, with support from exceptional faculty and bolstered by a world-class university, initiated significant changes aimed at building the future of dentistry based on innovation and scientific inquiry, not just for the school, but also for the entire oral health-care profession.

*Chapter 1*

# The Mann Years (1962–1981)

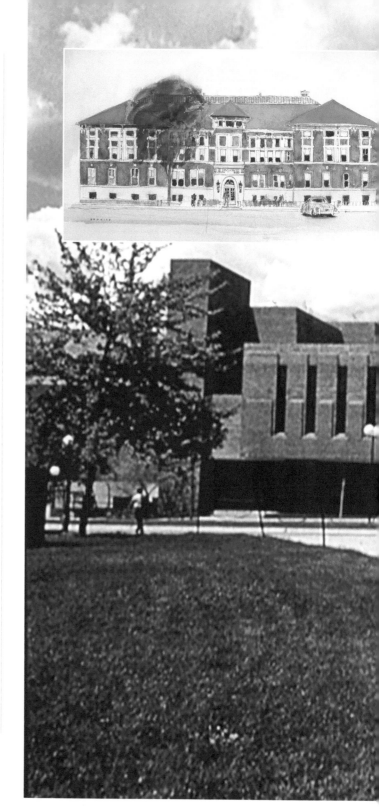

Dr. William Mann became dean on July 1, 1962. He brought to the position extensive experience as an administrator, teacher, and writer. Prior to his deanship, he held a half-time appointment with the American Council on Education as director of the Dental Education section and authored a 183-page report on dental education that was included in the final report—*The Survey of Dentistry: The Final Report*.[1] This national survey focused on dental health, dental practice, dental education, and dental research and had important implications for dental education and the profession of dentistry.[2]

## A Building for the Future

Perhaps the most visual symbol of the dramatic changes that occurred at the School of Dentistry during the five-and-a-half decades from 1962 to 2017 involved the construction of the new dental school building still in use today.

The need for a new facility was critical to the future of dental education at Michigan. The prospectus for the new building, dated February 12, 1964, was blunt in its assessment of the 1908 building. It stated:

The report on accreditation, made by the Council on Dental Education of the American

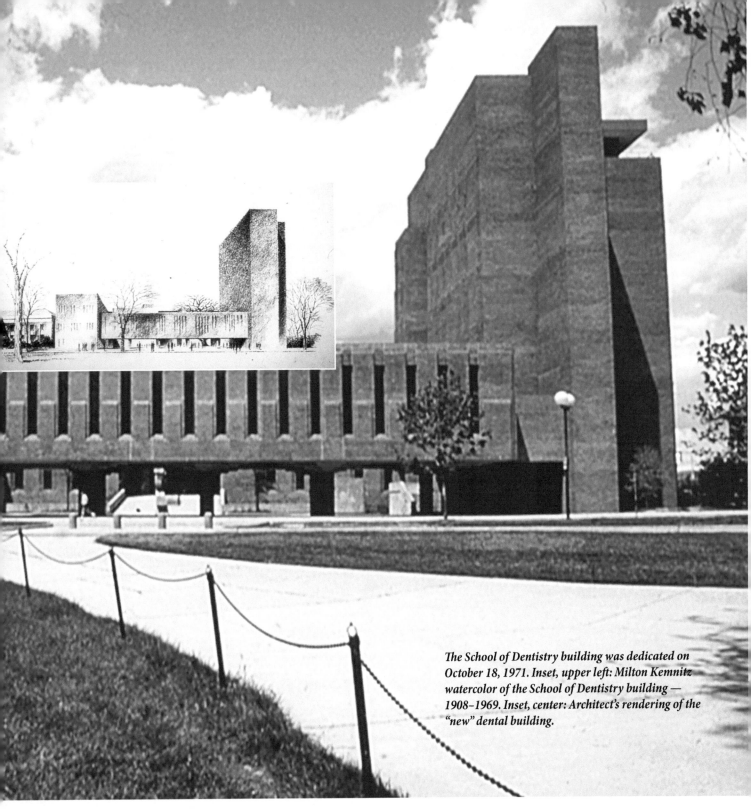

*The School of Dentistry building was dedicated on October 18, 1971. Inset, upper left: Milton Kemnitz watercolor of the School of Dentistry building — 1908-1969. Inset, center: Architect's rendering of the "new" dental building.*

Dental Association in 1961, noted that teaching facilities of the school fail to meet recommended standards for improved clinical and preclinical instruction. . . . Because of limited space the school has been unable to keep pace with the remarkable advances in dental education and research that have been made over the past 20 years. . . . The wholly inadequate research facilities now being used have been improvised from basement storage rooms. . . . Faculty must utilize locker space in the student locker room.[3]

In September 1962, Mann made an administrative appointment that, in hindsight, was crucial to the future of the School of Dentistry when he asked Dr. Robert Doerr to become associate dean. Doerr and Mann spent hundreds of hours with architects discussing in detail what facilities would be needed. Doerr also was instrumental in conducting a survey designed to project the future dental workforce needs of Michigan. Population forecasts and dental workforce data gathered from the survey further guided the planning and design process. Based on the results, it was determined that the new dental building

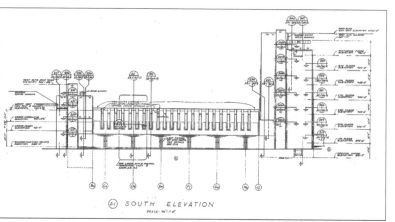

*Construction drawing, south elevation of the new Dental Building*

should have enough space to accommodate 150 dental students and 80 dental hygiene students in each class across the respective curricula.[4]

Designing a state-of-the-art facility to educate the leaders and best in dentistry was one thing, but funding this incredible undertaking was quite another. Funding commitments of $13 million from the State of Michigan, $5.6 million from the federal government, and $1.8 million from the Kellogg Foundation were obtained to cover construction costs.[5]

In "A Short History of the University of Michigan School of Dentistry" compiled by Charles Kelsey in 1971, Kelsey notes that the total cost of the dental school project was $17,294,855. At the time this was the largest building contract ever made in the history of the University of Michigan. By comparison, the cost to build the 1908 dental school building was $115,000. An addition to the facility in 1922–1923 totaled $128,000. The adjacent W.K. Kellogg Foundation Institute building was built in 1939–1940 for $450,000.[6]

Additional space was imperative if the School of Dentistry was going to be able to respond to the mandate to increase class size and advance the ever-growing research enterprise. The new dental complex offered significantly more space for all School of Dentistry activities. The 1908 building, including the later addition, was approximately 65,000 gross square feet. The W.K. Kellogg Foundation Institute building provided approximately 50,000 gross square feet. The new dental complex, when completed, would provide more than 293,300 gross square feet and when linked to the adjacent W.K. Kellogg Foundation Institute building would yield a total of 343,000 square feet to accommodate the growing teaching, research, patient care, and support services needs of the school.[6]

The design of the new dental complex consisted of four interconnected structures: the clinical wing (north), the research wing (east), the Kellogg wing (west), and the library (south). To minimize the impact on classroom instruction and clinical operations, the building project was staged in two phases: Phase I included the new clinical and research wings and Phase II included the Kellogg wing and the library.

With design completed and funding secured, construction officially commenced with the groundbreaking on February 2, 1966.

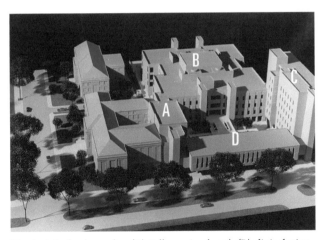

The dental school complex: (A) Kellogg wing (west), (B) clinical wing (north), (C) research wing (east), and (D) dental library (south).

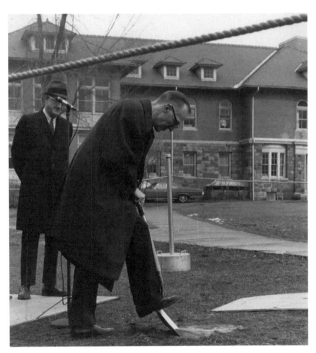

Dean William Mann turns the first shovel at the groundbreaking ceremony celebrating the start of construction of the new dental complex.

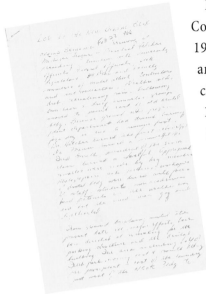

Dr. Frank Comstock (DDS 1950), professor and director of clinics (1969–1984), kept a handwritten log of some of the issues that occurred during the construction process. His log provides insight, from a faculty member's perspective, of what it was like to try to conduct business as usual with the seemingly endless thump of pile drivers as they worked to compress 60-foot tubes of steel into the ground for footings to support this enormous structure.[7]

## Construction Delays

In his log, Comstock noted that construction slowed in the spring of 1966 when excavation for the clinical wing and parking structure produced a massive hole that put the Health Services building in jeopardy.

Comstock wrote, "Troubles occurred in back of the H.S. where interlocking steel piling [sic] was driven and a retaining wall set up so the H.S would not slide into the excavation." A tradesmen's strike in early May stopped all work except for the emergency work needed to complete the retaining wall to stabilize the Health Services building.[8]

Comstock reported that by May 27, 1968, the skeleton of the new building was up with most work being completed inside. The parking structure was essentially finished, but the Fletcher Street entrance was not yet open. Comstock also commented on the Kellogg Foundation Institute's second summer of remodeling with floors being cut to install control boxes for new Ritter units

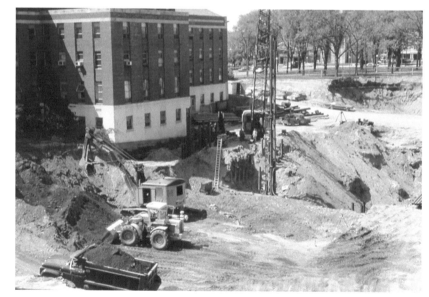

*Construction stopped while a retaining wall was built to stabilize the Health Services building.*

## An Unexpected Surprise

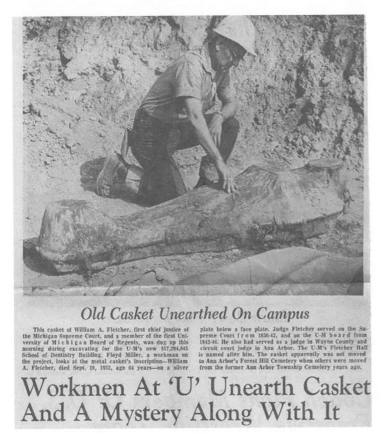

### Old Casket Unearthed On Campus

This casket of William A. Fletcher, first chief justice of the Michigan Supreme Court, and a member of the first University of Michigan Board of Regents, was dug up this morning during excavating for the U-M's new $17,291,845 School of Dentistry Building. Floyd Miller, a workman on the project, looks at the metal casket's inscription—William A. Fletcher, died Sept. 19, 1852, age 64 years—on a silver plate below a face plate. Judge Fletcher served on the Supreme Court from 1836-42, and on the U-M board from 1842-46. He also had served as a judge in Wayne County and circuit court judge in Ann Arbor. The U-M's Fletcher Hall is named after him. The casket apparently was not moved to Ann Arbor's Forest Hill Cemetery when others were moved from the former Ann Arbor Township Cemetery years ago.

# Workmen At 'U' Unearth Casket And A Mystery Along With It

*From the* Ann Arbor News, *June 6, 1966. Reprinted with permission from the Ann Arbor News.*

On June 6, 1966, workmen excavating along the northwest corner of the dental complex construction site were surprised when they dug up a metal casket. Presumably, the casket contained the remains of William A. Fletcher, chief justice of the Michigan Supreme Court and a member of the U-M's first Board of Regents, who died September 19, 1852. Fletcher, who also had served as a circuit judge in Ann Arbor, was buried in the Ann Arbor Township Cemetery. That cemetery, now Felch Park, located on the corner of Huron and Fletcher Streets was abandoned in 1918 and all caskets were moved to Forest Hill Cemetery off of Geddes Avenue.[9] All caskets save one, the one the workers uncovered. The Comstock notes dated June 7, 1966 quipped, "Rumor circulated that the casket was filled with alcohol. If so, one can assume he was pickled for 114 years which could be a record."

scheduled to be installed sometime after June 1, 1968. He concluded this entry with the comment that they "continue to be plagued by labor unrest."

Labor issues and strikes were responsible for numerous delays throughout the final year and a half of construction.

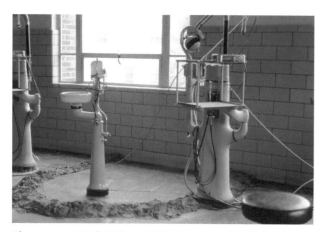

*Floors were cut in the Kellogg Building in preparation for the installation of new dental units.*

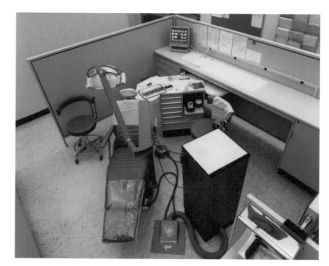

*One of the 36 cubicles set up and ready for patient care.*

## Phase I Finished

Everyone was thrilled when Phase I was completed in August 1969, and classes and clinic operations moved into the new structure for the beginning of the fall semester.

The new clinical wing served as the main instructional facility. This five-story structure featured the very latest in clinical equipment and instructional technology. The basement housed the building's services. Three 156-seat lecture halls, a seminar room, preclinical laboratories, student locker room, and student lobby occupied the ground floor. Preclinical laboratories, where first- and second-year dental students learned the foundations of clinical procedures and techniques, occupied approximately 7,700 square feet.

Clinics were located on the first, second, and third floors. First floor clinics included oral diagnosis,

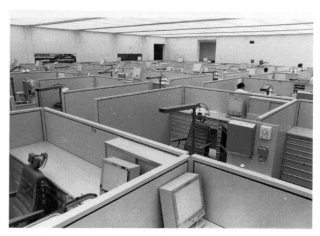

*Cubicle layout in the new clinical wing.*

radiology, pediatric dentistry, periodontics and periodontal surgery, crown and bridge, and dental auxiliary utilization. The main dental laboratory was also housed on this level. The senior clinic was located

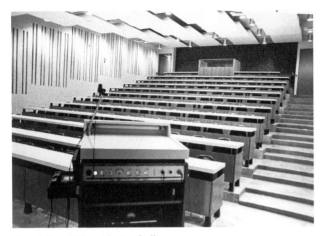

One of three 156-seat lecture halls.

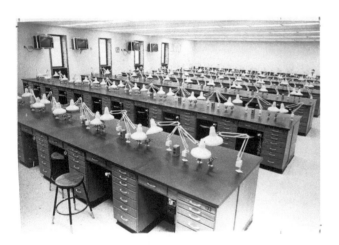

The preclinical laboratory on the east side of the ground floor of the new dental building. A second preclinical laboratory was located on the west side.

on the second floor. This clinic was divided into four quadrants, each with 36 individually partitioned operatories for patient privacy. Each of the four clinic quadrants had slightly more than 4,000 square feet of space. The junior clinics, general clinics, and the central records room were located on the third floor. The central records room housed both the school's computing unit and an automatic patient record retrieval system.

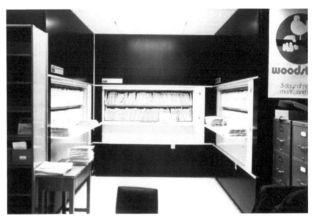

The central records room featured an automatic patient record retrieval system.

## The Research Tower

The adjacent nine-story research wing, which over the years became known as the "Research Tower," also was ready for occupancy in 1969.[10] Administrative offices were located on the ground and first floors with the second through sixth floors dedicated to much needed research space as well as offices for the faculty scientist. Laboratory space in the Research Tower added 21,000 square feet, a crucial addition to the school's growing research enterprise. The seventh

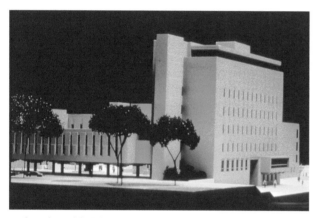

*Architect's model of the seven-story Research Tower on the east side of the new dental building complex.*

floor housed the Faculty Alumni Lounge that provided space for meetings, conferences, and events. Generous contributions from alumni donors were designated to purchase the furnishings for the Faculty Alumni Lounge.

With the successful move into the new clinical wing, demolition of the 1908 dental school structure commenced along with site preparation and construction of the Kellogg wing and the library—Phase II of the construction plan.

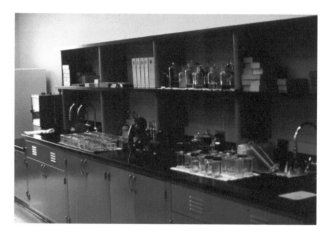

*One of the many new research laboratories in the new Research Tower.*

## Phase II Finished

Phase II projects of the new dental complex were completed in 1971. The dental library, a divisional library of the U-M Library, was built on the site of the 1908 dental building and opened for general use in June 1971.[11,12] For the two years the library

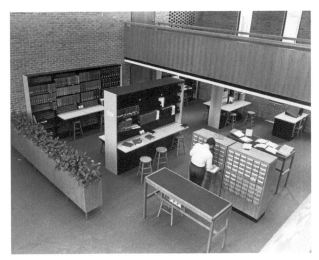

*Students and faculty have ready access to reference and resource materials.*

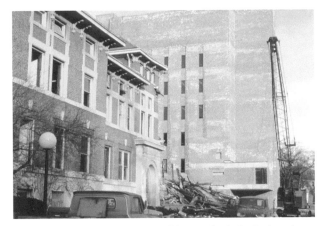

*The demolition of the old dental building marks the beginning of Phase II of construction.*

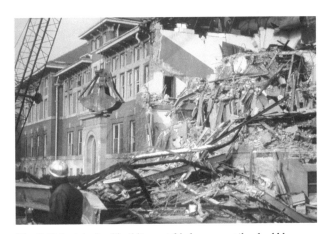

*The 1908 dental school building quickly became a pile of rubble.*

was under construction, all of its holdings were located in temporary facilities in the basement of the new clinical wing. Faculty and students were thrilled when they could, once again, easily access more than 46,000 items available for circulation and 28,000 copies of reserve materials in the spacious, two-story building.[11] The library became increasingly recognized as one of the finest and most complete dentistry libraries in the world.

A special enhancement to the teaching program was an instructional television center, located on the third floor of the Kellogg wing. This facility became operational in the fall of 1971 with the help of alumni donors who stepped up and provided funds to assist with the purchase of video equipment for the center, creating a state-of-the-art television studio.

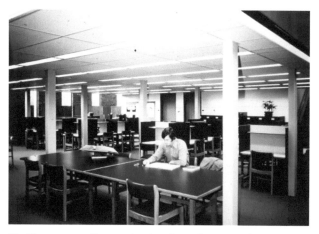

*The library space offers a quiet place for students to study.*

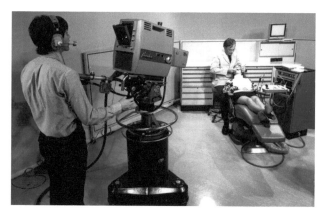

*Filming dental procedures help enhance student learning.*

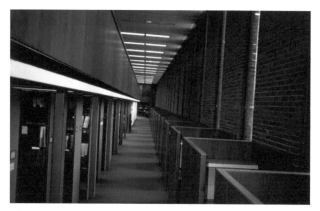

*There are plenty of study carrels in the new library.*

The 1,800-square-foot studio was the site where thousands of videotapes on oral health topics and dental procedures were produced and used extensively to educate U-M School of Dentistry students. The videotapes also were distributed to other dental schools and health organizations around the world. As new technology evolved, so did the capability of this facility.

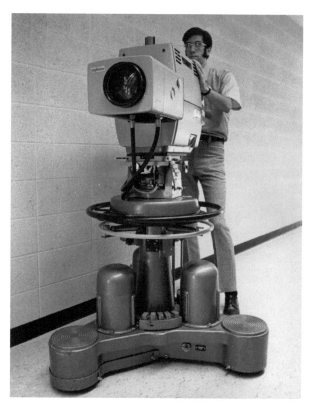

*Howard Mevis with one of the TV cameras. Portable cameras could be easily moved about the building to film in many different locations.*

Many of these historic videos still are available for viewing today on the U-M Dentistry YouTube channel.[13]

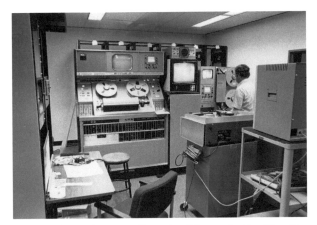

*A state-of- the-art television studio produced thousands of teaching videos.*

## Open House

Before unveiling the new building to the public, dental school administrators held an open house on Sunday, October 3, 1971. In his September newsletter to the school's faculty and staff, Mann wrote:

> Essentially we will be showing off the new facilities; but since they are designed as a setting for modern dental education, we will also be putting the nature of modern dentistry and dental research on display, a thing which is in our interest to do well and to the best advantage. [He expressed his desire] to have all activities staffed and open to view in such a way as to give an impression of the school as it is on a normal class day.[14]

## Dedication

The official dedication of the new dental complex was held on October 18, 1971, marking the most significant milestone in the School of Dentistry's history. As Mann cut the symbolic ribbon opening the new dental complex, he said that the new facility would allow the school to admit more students to study dentistry and dental hygiene and that

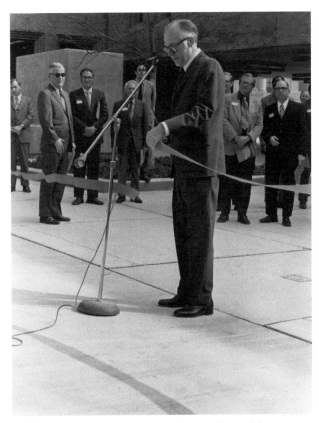

*The ribbon cutting ceremony marking the completion of the new dental complex was held on October, 18, 1971.*

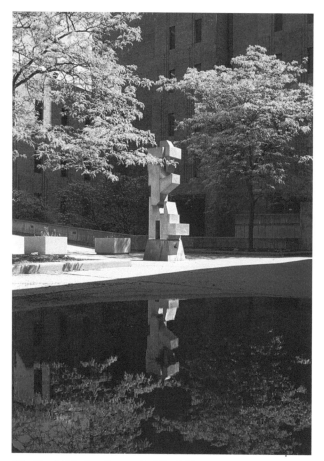

*"The Tooth Fairy" sculpture off of North University Avenue at the main entrance to the School of Dentistry.*

That same day, a sculpture was unveiled on the plaza adjacent to North University Avenue entrance. A gift from the Class of 1944, the irregularly shaped aluminum sculpture was created by Bill Barrett, a well-known local artist who later moved to New York City. "The sculpture has no title, nor any abstract relation to dentistry or any other subject or object. It does not 'represent.' Instead it is an object designed for its place," Mann wrote. Over the years, however, the sculpture has been often referred to as "The Tooth Fairy."[15]

Although the sculptor said the piece was merely an object designed for its place, to the trained eye of many dental professional, it looks to have incorporated the many angles and cuts used in dentistry to create restorative preparations.

## Mixed Reactions

The clean lines of the Modernist architecture prominent in structures built in the 1960s and reflected in the esthetics of the new dental complex were disconcerting to some.

Henry Kanar (MS Pediatric Dentistry 1971), a faculty member from 1971 to 1998, remembers overhearing faculty, who repeatedly emphasized the importance of precision in dentistry, jest that "not all the building's bricks were in a straight line."

changes and improvements in the curriculum would now be possible. Those words launched amazing transformations in dental education at U-M that for decades to come would be recognized as a gold standard for curriculum design and educational innovation.

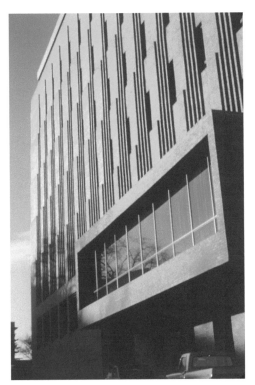

*Straight lines were a prominent architectural feature on the new building's exterior.*

Jack Gobetti (DDS 1968, MS Oral Diagnosis and Radiology 1971), a dental school faculty member for more than 40 years, spent most of his dental school years in the old building. Gobetti thought the new building was a little stark: "The old dental school building had personality and charm with its beautiful wood, brass railings and other features."

Richard Johnson (DDS 1967, MS Orthodontics 1973), a faculty member for more than 30 years, shared similar feelings: "There was something about the old building that really made it stand out. . . . Foremost, in my mind, was the beautiful wood paneling. It conveyed sophistication and class.

Architectural issues aside, the new building offered students, faculty, and staff much needed space to teach, learn, and deliver state-of-the-art dental care. It also enabled the school to increase class size to address the expected shortages in the dental workforce.

**The Paul Bunyan Murals:** Another important element of the old building's warmth, according to some, was in the pediatric dental clinic

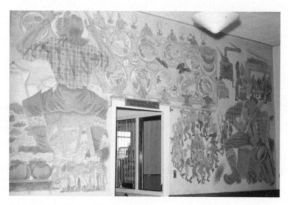

*One wall of the Paul Bunyan mural outside the orthodontic clinic in the old dental building.*

where images depicting the life of the legendary lumberjack, Paul Bunyan, and his companion, Babe the Blue Ox, were prominently displayed. The characters were painted by artist Francis Danovich after being commissioned by the U.S. Works Progress Administration in 1939. Children gravitated to the mural because of its size and the colors. Parents also enjoyed the mural and became involved as they answered their children's questions about the whimsical life of the legendary lumberman and his friends.[16]

The mural, however, was covered by wallpaper during the 1970s and was all but forgotten. It was "rediscovered" during renovations to the Kellogg Building in 1999. By that time, though, several sections of the original mural had been damaged and only portions of the mural could be salvaged. The mural sections that were salvaged were framed and relocated to the Sindecuse Museum Atrium (Ann Arbor, MI) where they reside today.

## Projecting Dental Workforce Needs

Foremost among the projections was a sharp rise in population. As a manufacturing state whose employers offered good wages and fringe benefits, Michigan was a magnet that attracted men and women from across the nation to work for auto companies and many of their suppliers. In 1970, the state's population was approximately 8.9 million, an increase of more than 13 percent from 1960. That percentage growth rate matched the growth rate of the U.S. population when the nation's headcount rose from 179.32 million in 1960 to 203.2 million by 1970.[17] By 1980, the state's population increased nearly 4.5 percent to 9.26 million.[18]

During this time, the growth of auto manufacturing and membership in labor unions (where nearly 30 percent of wage and salary workers belonged to a union) resulted in a demand not just for higher wages, but also for fringe benefits, including a new one—dental care—which, in turn, led to increased demand for oral health-care professionals. "Union contract negotiations are now heading toward incorporation of dental service as a fringe benefit. Such a fringe benefit will increase the demand for dentists," according to minutes of an April 13, 1973, meeting of the U-M's Office of Capital Planning, whose members met with School of Dentistry administrators to discuss the school's needs. Minutes from the same meeting noted, "there is a possibility of a tremendous increase in demand for dental care. In the neighborhood of only 40–50 percent of the population now sees a dentist each year."[19]

## The Need for More Dental Health Professionals

The American Dental Association (ADA) reported there were 4,734 dentists in Michigan in 1970. The U-M Long-Range Planning Subcommittee on School and College Planning met with the School of Dentistry leadership on December 1, 1972, to review population and workforce data in Michigan. The dentist-to-population numbers presented showed "the ratio in Michigan is 1 dentist for every 1,850 population compared to the national ratio of 1:1,683."[20] A shortage of dentists in Michigan was looming.

The impetus to increase the number of dental students graduating from the U-M School of Dentistry also was driven by fears about the long-term viability of the state's other dental school. According to minutes from that same December 1972 meeting,

> The University of Detroit Dental School is in financial trouble . . . U of D administrators feel that their dental school can last approximately five years. . . . Legislators are worried about the impact of these trends, and are working with the dean and the Executive Committee to plan for the state's dental needs in the next ten to fifteen years. [20]

## Dental and Dental Hygiene Enrollments

From the mid-1940s through the opening of the new dental building in 1971, first-year dental class enrollment averaged 90 students per year. As had been planned, the additional space, both classroom and clinic, in the new building allowed the school to increase the doctor of dental surgery (DDS) and dental hygiene class sizes. By the mid-1970s, first-year enrollment in the dental program increased to more than 150 students with largest class of 154 students admitted in 1975.[21]

Throughout the 1970s and into the early1980s, the number of graduating dental students ranged from a low of 83 in 1971 to a peak of 151 graduates in 1978.

Opening the new dental building in 1971 was a milestone for the dental hygiene program. The annual admissions cap of 39, necessitated by severe space limitations, was raised to 80. The program maintained that class size until 1980.[21,22]

**DDS Admission Data 1970–1980**

| Students entering the fall of: | Total Admitted* |
|---|---|
| 1970 | 132 |
| 1971 | 135 |
| 1972 | 150 |
| 1973 | 152 |
| 1974 | 151 |
| 1975 | 154 |
| 1976 | 152 |
| 1977 | 151 |
| 1978 | 151 |
| 1979 | 151 |
| 1980 | 151 |

\* Information retrieved from admissions files archived in the School of Dentistry's Office of Admissions.

**DDS Graduation Data 1970–1980**

| Year of Graduation | Total DDS Graduates* |
|---|---|
| 1970 | 92 |
| 1971 | 83 |
| 1972 | 100 |
| 1973 | 117 |
| 1974 | 122 |
| 1975 | 140 |
| 1976 | 136 |
| 1977 | 149 |
| 1978 | 151 |
| 1979 | 139 |
| 1980 | 140 |

\* Information retrieved from admissions files archived in the School of Dentistry's Office of Admissions.

Students entering the dental hygiene curriculum in the 1970s were enrolled in either a two-year program or a four-year program. The two-year curriculum was designed to train women to become dental hygienists. A limited number of students were admitted as freshmen directly from high school each fall. After successfully completing the program, they received a certificate in dental hygiene. The four-year curriculum consisted of two years of liberal arts education followed by two years of dental hygiene study at the School of Dentistry. The four-year program was designed for those who wanted to prepare themselves to become teachers or leaders in the dental hygiene profession. At graduation,

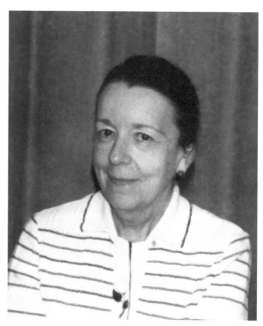

*Pauline Steele, director of dental hygiene, 1968–1988.*

students received a Bachelor of Science degree in dental hygiene.[21]

Under the leadership of Pauline Steele, director of the dental hygiene program 1968–1988, the number of dental hygiene students graduating with either a certificate or a bachelor's degree increased from 38 graduates per year in 1970 to 79 per year in 1980.

The significant increases in the number of dental and dental hygiene students enrolled in a degree or certificate program at the School of Dentistry was expected. Both school and U-M leaders, who in the years leading up to the groundbreaking for the school's new facilities, had carefully researched projections related to population growth and health-care workforce trends in Michigan and across the nation.

Total enrollment for all groups, including graduate programs, increased markedly from 1970 to 1979. The school enrolled 669 students at the start of the 1970 academic year. By the 1979 academic year, the total enrollment number had increased to 849 students across all programs. During this time period, the enrollment numbers peaked in 1976 when total enrollment for all programs reached 854 and the four DDS classes totaled 602. The master's program experienced a dramatic rise in 1979.[22]

### Student Enrollment Comparison: 1970–1979

| Year | Total | DDS | DH | Master's | PhD |
|------|-------|-----|-----|----------|-----|
| 1970 | 669 | 441 | 134 | 89 | 5 |
| 1979 | 849 | 591 | 157 | 100 | 1 |

## Health Professions Educational Assistance

To help meet the growing demand for dentists, physicians, and other health professionals, Congress enacted the Health Professions Educational Assistance Act in 1963. The act authorized two significant initiatives. The first was a construction grant assistance program to help build new facilities to increase capacity for schools of medicine, dentistry, osteopathy, optometry, pharmacy, podiatry, public health, and professional nursing. The second important initiative was a student loan program to help talented, but needy students afford the significant costs associated with pursuing a career in the health professions.

After the act was passed, the U.S. Public Health Service advised Congress that the nation faced a severe shortage of approximately 17,800 dentists during the 1970s. "While these figures are most astounding, the projected shortages for 1980 are even more frightening. Based on present policy trends, manpower shortages for the end of this decade are expected to number 56,600 dentists," the U.S. Public Health Service noted in a report. Congress amended the act several times following passage in 1963 with some of the most extensive additions and modifications made in the passage of the Comprehensive Health Manpower Training Act of 1971.[23] This act raised incentives for increasing enrollments and graduates, and shifted emphasis from construction support to institutional support to schools.

## Capitation Grants

Important to the School of Dentistry was a major new provision in the 1971 act, per capita assistance, more commonly referred to as "capitation grants." These grants were awarded based on a headcount of students with the goal to help schools stabilize their finances. The grants also were designed to help dental, medical, and other health-care schools attract students who, after graduation, could meet the growing demand for dental and other health-care services in areas of need, especially rural communities and inner cities.

In a letter dated April 25, 1972 to U-M Vice President for Academic Affairs Allan Smith, Dean Mann outlined the school's financial picture and concluded, "The School of Dentistry is deeply dependent upon the funds which will be provided by the 1972–73 capitation grant in order to carry on its programs." The amount cited in the letter was $1 million.[24] On August 8, in another memo to Smith, Mann advised the school was awarded a capitation grant of $1,047,869 for the 1972–1973 academic year. He also noted a "bonus class" clause in the capitation grant language. "This means that for the next three years, or four, if similar legislation is continued, we will receive $150,000 more than we were entitled to on the basis of enrollment only."[25]

An important provision of the 1971 act was awarding education grants to students enrolled in schools of dentistry, medicine, osteopathy, and other health professions. Per-student grants of $2,500 were awarded for full-time first-, second-, or third-year students. The amount increased to $4,000 for fourth-year students. The act also provided for partial loan forgiveness to students if they worked in areas, such as rural areas and inner cities, where there were health-care workforce shortages. Loan forgiveness totaled 30 percent each year for the first two years of service and 25 percent for the third year. It also allowed public and private nonprofit schools of dentistry, medicine, osteopathy, veterinary medicine, public health, pharmacy, podiatry, or a combination of those schools to apply for construction grant assistance.[26]

## Dental School Funding

The School of Dentistry pursued a two-track strategy. The first was to take advantage of federal legislation. The second was to work with top U-M administrators and state legislators in Lansing to try to obtain additional state funding to run the dental school.

First-year dental student enrollment increased from 132 in 1970 to 152 in 1973. An additional increase to 165 was proposed for 1975. Concern was expressed among School of Dentistry administrators that the number of first-year dental students would continue to increase beyond 151 students. Just two years after the new dental school building opened, minutes from the April 13, 1973, budget meeting show Mann advising: "The school's dental facilities were built for the present class size of 150. The (proposed) increase to 165 (first-year dental students) in 1975 will cause some overcrowding."[27]

In a seven-page letter to U-M Vice President of Academic Affairs Frank Rhodes dated January 6, 1975, Mann reported:

> When funds for its new building were approved, the School agreed to expand the size of its student body. Fortunately, during the past several years the School of Dentistry has been successful in persuading the State Legislature to appropriate annual increases for its operating budget which were large enough to permit the school to fund its programs reasonably well as its enrollment increased. In addition, for the past two years, the school has received a sizable amount of money from the federal government in the form of a "capitation grant" that could be used for operating purposes as related to the DDS program. [28]

On page 2 of that letter, Mann included this phrase: "*the line item appropriation for the School of Dentistry.*" Those nine words were revealing.

Typically, a single-dollar amount labeled "University of Michigan–Ann Arbor" was noted in the state budget. However, from 1970 through 1985, instead of being lumped into the university's total budget, the state specifically set aside funds for the School of Dentistry as a separate line item for two of its crucial functions. One was for administration and operations and the other to help cope with increases in class size.

Jed Jacobson (DDS 1978), former faculty member who served as assistant dean for admissions as well as assistant dean for community and outreach programs, said: "We as faculty members knew about the line item in the state budget for the school." The significance was lost on no one because the School of Dentistry having

| PUBLIC ACTS 1975—No. 263 | | 1011 |
|---|---|---|
| | | For Fiscal Year Ending June 30, 1976 |

entering class of 151 and a total undergraduate enrollment of 596 in 1975-76, and an entering class of 151 and total undergraduate enrollment of 608 in 1976-77, also including $76,100 for expanded duty auxiliary program.) .......... $ 171,968,700
In-state student fees ................................. 24,748,000
Out-of-state student fees ........................... 20,962,000
Off-campus student fees ............................ 1,190,000
Other income ......................................... 16,366,600
Total institutional revenues ................... $ 63,266,600

In recognition of the aforementioned financial needs and institutional sources of operating revenue, there is appropriated to the university of Michigan—Ann Arbor from the general fund of the state for fiscal year ending June 30, 1976, the following respective amounts for the following purposes:

Instruction

| | |
|---|---|
| Architecture and design (767 CYES) ................. $ | 1,734,900 |
| Business administration (1,453 CYES) ................. | 2,052,000 |
| Dentistry (including $137,300 for continuing expansion to an entering class of 151 and a total undergraduate enrollment of 596 in 1975-76 and an entering class of 151 and total undergraduate enrollment of 608 in 1976-77, also including $76,100 for expanded duty auxiliary program.) (806 CYES) ................. | 5,005,400 |
| Education (2,184 CYES) ................................. | 2,197,700 |
| Engineering (2,595 CYES) .............................. | 6,231,200 |
| Graduate school ........................................ | 656,200 |
| Law school (1,226 CYES) ............................... | 1,381,900 |
| Library science (320 CYES) ............................ | 322,800 |
| Literature, science and arts (18,368 CYES) ........... | 16,971,200 |
| Medical school (including an entering class of 202 and a total undergraduate enrollment of 925 in 1975-76 and an entering class of 202 and a total undergraduate enrollment of 925 in 1976-77, and $533,900 for continuing expansion to an entering class of 50 inteflex students and a total undergraduate inteflex enrollment of 180 in 1975-76, and an entering inteflex class of 50 and a total undergraduate inteflex enrollment of 217 in 1976-77) (3,063 CYES) ................. | 9,401,800 |
| Mental health units .................................... | 8,318,500 |
| Music (972 CYES) ...................................... | 2,017,000 |
| Natural resources (654 CYES) ......................... | 1,513,200 |
| Nursing (628 CYES) .................................... | 1,269,600 |
| Pharmacy (215 CYES) .................................. | 492,600 |

*Page 1011 from Public Acts 1975–No. 263 for fiscal year ending June 30, 1976, specifying special appropriations for the School of Dentistry.*

a separate line item appropriation in the state budget meant that vital funds were being given to the school to support the demands of DDS program.

In 1970, for example, the state specifically approved a $3.8-million appropriation "for administration and operation of the dental school." An additional $497,400 was set aside "for expansion to 130 (entering) class level." In 1971, $4.4 million was listed in the state budget for administration and operation of the dental school and another $320,000 appropriated to expand the size of the first-year dental class to 145 students. From 1970 to 1975, the school received nearly $1.8 million in additional appropriations to enable it to enroll more dental students. Between 1970 and 1985, the school received more than $97.6 million for administration and operations. Separately, between 1970 and 1975, nearly $1.8 million more was appropriated to allow the school to increase enrollment to accommodate 130, 145, 150, and ultimately 151 first-year dental students.[29]

## Curriculum Review

Periodic curriculum review is essential in dental education. As research informs dental practice, then products, techniques, and technology must be taught to the students and the dental curriculum must adapt.

In 1962, the school's Committee on Curriculum conducted a comprehensive review and began designing a progressive new dental program to graduate practitioners possessing the skills, competencies, and intellectual adaptability to cope with both present and future requirements of oral health care and practice.

The committee sought opinions from faculty, students, and alumni in 1964 and 1965. In August 1967, a faculty conference was conducted in Ann Arbor, at which time details of the new dental curriculum were presented to the dental faculty and to members of the basic science departments of the Medical School who taught dental students. The faculty adopted the new curriculum that was launched in the fall of 1969 and coincided with the opening of the clinical wing of the new dental complex.[30]

The new DDS curriculum was designed for flexibility to accommodate changing concepts in how dentistry was practiced and focused on the activities and initiatives of the 18 different departments within the school. Those departments (in alphabetical order) were as follows: Community Dentistry, Complete Denture Prosthodontics, Crown and Bridge Prosthesis, Dental Materials, Dentistry in the University Hospital, Educational Resources, Endodontics, Occlusion, Operative Dentistry, Oral Biology, Oral Diagnosis and Radiology, Oral Pathology, Oral Surgery, Orthodontics, Partial Denture Prosthodontics, Pedodontics, Periodontics, and Preclinical Dentistry.[30]

## New Technology Enhances Curriculum

In an annual report to the president of U-M for the 1977–1978 academic year, Mann noted that nearly 350 television recording and editing sessions had been conducted and "playbacks of tapes to classrooms and duplications (of those videotapes) for local and international distribution reached their highest level (3,908) since the school's inauguration of television use in 1970."[31] Under the direction of Dr. David Starks,

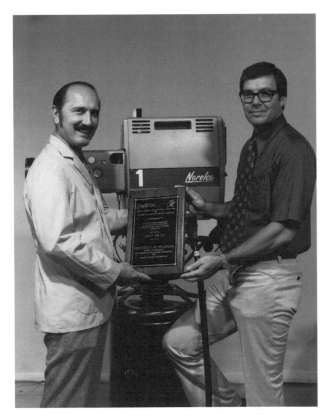

*In 1975, the Department of Educational Resources won first prize from the Health Sciences Communications Association and the Network for Continuing Medical Education for the use of television for education in the health sciences. Holding the plaque are Dr. Robert Lowery (L) and Mr. Charles Eddlemon.*

chair of the Department of Educational Resources, who assumed his duties in July 1972, original photography, film processing and printing, and television and video production were done in-house by the department's staff.[32]

## Building the Video Library

For more than 20 years, the staff in the Department of Educational Resources worked closely with the faculty to incorporate photography, videography, and dental and medical illustration into the curriculum to enhance learning. Many of the lectures and demonstrations transmitted to classrooms and laboratories via the school's television studio were captured on videotape.

In a July 17, 1984 memo to the school's Budget Priorities Committee Starks noted:

> Since the early 1970s, the contributions of television to the quality of dental teaching have been widely recognized. . . . Faculty have adopted television into their teaching to such an extent that, on average, each student views one videotape per day throughout most semesters.

Noting that "more than 1,000 tapes in our current library" were produced between 1972 and 1984, Stark added that "faculty at schools throughout the country and around the world are looking to Michigan to supply tapes for teaching in a variety of fields." He also noted sales of the videotapes provided income for the school that ranged from $14,000 to $60,000 annually. Ultimately, nearly 2,000 videotapes related to a host of dental topics covering clinical and laboratory procedures were produced in the television studios on the third floor.

In July 1972, the school received a $700,000 federal grant to establish a pilot program in dental education that allowed students to advance through the dental curriculum at their own individual rate of

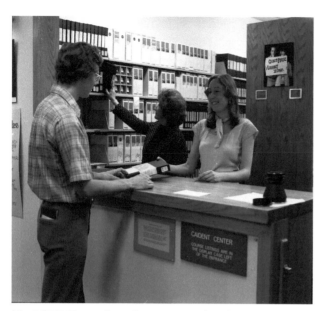

*The CAIDENT center housed course materials and other learning resources used by the students.*

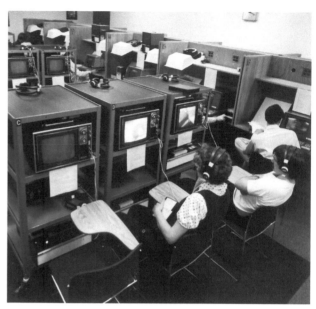

*Students accessed audio-visual study materials in the CAIDENT center.*

learning. Funds were used to construct an independent learning center, known as CAIDENT (Computer-Aided Instruction DENTistry). The library-like facility, located in the basement of the new dental building, occupied about 2,400 square feet of floor area and provided instructional materials to students and faculty that included videotapes of lectures captured in the television studio, 35-mm slides, audiocassettes, or printed handouts.[33] It also had an audio engineering studio where faculty often narrated scripts they wrote to accompany a lecture or technique they were teaching.

## Keeping Pace with Technology

John Squires, whose 35-year career at U-M included 33 years at the School of Dentistry, remembers his first day as a TV video engineer. "I was riding the elevator with Dr. John Lillie, an anatomist and cell biologist, who was holding a container," Squires said. "When I asked him what was inside, he removed the lid and showed me a human head. I nearly fainted before we got

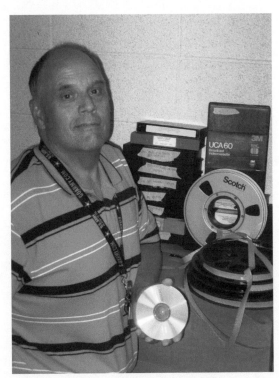

*John Squires retired as chief media engineer in 2013.*

off the elevator which was near the third-floor television studios," he added. The head was used to videotape a lecture on head and neck anatomy.

He was hired in the late 1970s to manage the equipment in the CAIDENT center. During the mid-1980s, he became the chief media engineer and redesigned and rebuilt the school's television studio to include state-of-the-art television cameras and videotape recorders. "We produced dozens of videos a month that were in high demand not only because of our reputation for quality production, but also because of the stellar reputation of our faculty and the information they presented," Squires said.

As technology advanced, Squires devoted more time and attention to personal computers and computer programming. He said when Starks purchased an Apple computer and a laser printer and brought them to the school, "I was hooked." Squires used his technical talents to link several dozen computers, so their users could communicate throughout the School of Dentistry on what became known as the "Apple Talk Network." The network was later replaced with faster Ethernet connections. With the growing use of computers and the World Wide Web, those videotapes would continue being used, although in new ways, in the twenty-first century.

## Behind the Camera

Per Kjeldsen, a photographer at the School of Dentistry for more than 32 years, said the school's embracing of new technology "was one of the major reasons I came to Michigan from the Rochester (New York) Institute of Technology." When he arrived at U-M in 1974, the school was developing self-instructional materials for education and research, and photography was an important part of those materials. "I wanted to be involved in those efforts," he said.

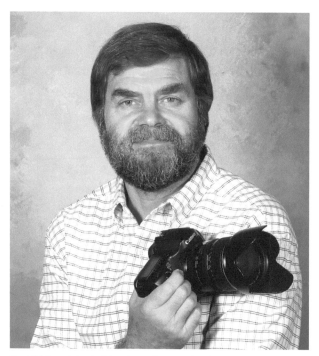

*Per Kjeldsen, School of Dentistry photographer from 1974–2006.*

As chief photographer from 1974 until 2006, Kjeldsen probably met, even if for only a few moments, every dental and dental hygiene student as he was taking their individual portraits for a composite class picture. It is also safe to say that he has met every dean, every administrator, every faculty member, and nearly every staff member as well. It is a claim few can make.[34]

Although he has photographed many school events, Kjeldsen says:

> [Graduation] is one event that hasn't changed over the years, and that's a good thing! The pride and joy that is reflected in the faces of the students, their parents and instructors is wonderful. I feel privileged to have captured so many of these special moments. (Personal communication, August 21, 2015)

During the pre-digital age, producing the class composites was a laborious work of art. After taking photos of all the students, the individual portraits were manually attached to an oversized board that Kjeldsen then sent to Florida. There, a calligrapher inscribed the

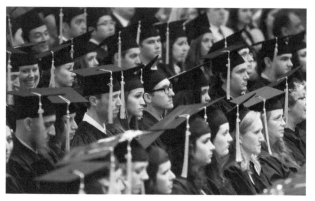

*Graduation 2012.*

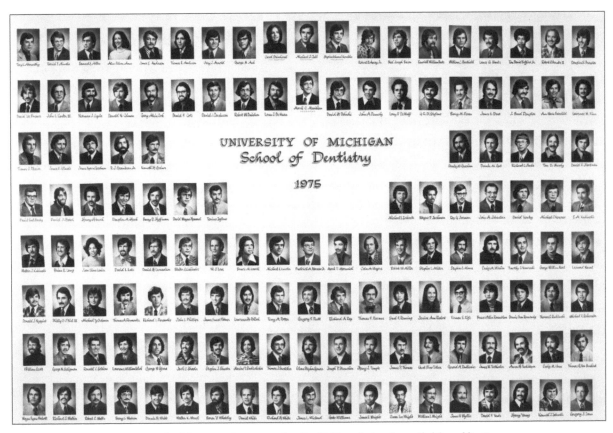

*The Class of 1975 is just one example of the many class composites Per Kjeldsen shot and compiled for publication.*

name of each dental class and each dental student. The finished board was then shipped back to Ann Arbor and a large negative was made of the board with all the photos and student names. Today, computer software makes producing both the class composites and the graduation composites much easier. The graduation composites of all of the dental and dental hygiene classes dating back to the very first DDS class are on display along the ground floor hallways near the lecture halls and in the Alpha Omega Student Forum.

## Professionalism and Appearance

When he began his teaching career at the School of Dentistry in 1970, Dr. Richard Johnson said "there was an aura of professionalism that permeated the school because of the dress code." Perhaps the most apparent feature of the dress code "was that men had to wear a sport coat and tie, and women had to wear dresses. "To many, appearance mattered since it conveyed the professionalism of the dental profession," he added.

As the decade of the 1960s gave way to the decade of the 1970s, fashions transitioned to a blend of hippie chic and bohemian mod. The clothing worn by dental students became a significant concern for many administrators and faculty who felt the attire seen throughout the dental school was sliding.

The front page of the March 18, 1970, issue of a school newsletter, *SSF Relater: A Publication by and for Students, Staff and Faculty*, reported, "The issue of student dress and appearance was discussed at several faculty meetings and at meetings within each department."

The article continued:

> The matter of appearance is of great importance to the dental profession. The maintenance of respect of as much of the population as possible is vital to keep the confidence of the people and as a result continue the service on a high level. To a large segment of the population, the matter of appearance seems to play a major role in personal evaluation.[35]

By the mid-1970s, the dress code had been relaxed considerably. Jed Jacobson (DDS 1978) said "we were not wearing ties in 1974 when I began my dental education."

## Guidelines for Student Appearance

### The University of Michigan School of Dentistry

1. *Clinic Floors:* Clinic coats must be worn while treating patients. Clinic coats or shirt and tie with lab coat must be worn while observing patient treatment or while doing lab work.

2. *Ground Floor and Basement:* Dress shirt, sport shirt, or turtleneck may be worn in labs and lecture rooms.

3. Clean, pressed slacks must be worn during clinic hours. (No Levis or extreme slacks.) Clean and neat footwear is required.

4. Students' hair should be neat and clean. In clinic situations, students' hair should not break the chain of asepsis nor interfere with clinical performance. No beards. Hair should not drape over the collar.

5. Clinic and lab coats are not to be worn outside the building. Clinic coats should not be worn during lectures.

6. Rules in effect from 8:00 A.M. to 5:00 P.M., Monday through Friday, and Saturday morning.

*Source:* Published in the *SSF Relater: A Publication by and for Students, Staff and Faculty* (March 18, 1970).

The importance of personal appearance as well as posture had long been emphasized in the dental hygiene program as well. Former students still have vivid recollections of Dr. Dorothy Hard, dental hygiene director 1928–1968, and the emphasis she placed on neatness and appearance. Two women graduates of the first class of the school's Master of Science in dental hygiene program, Karen Ross Peterson and Sandra Sonner Klinesteker, clearly remember Hard's sage counsel.

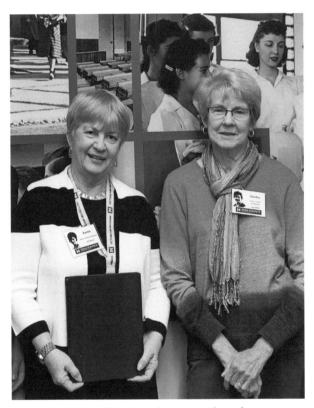

*Karen Ross Peterson (R) and Sandra Sonner Klinesteker were among the first graduates of the Master of Science in Dental Hygiene program. Peterson is holding her master's thesis published in 1965.*

Peterson recalled, "Dr. Hard presented herself very professionally and expected us to do the same." Klinesteker agreed, adding, "Dr. Hard always emphasized the importance of appearance because it conveyed professionalism." Klinesteker also remembered Hard's emphasis on keeping one's fingernails trimmed to reduce the risk of bacterial infection. Klinesteker said with a laugh:

> She told us our nails had to be short enough so that when we held up our hands, palms facing us, we couldn't see our nails. Of course, we didn't wear gloves at that time. But we did wear a white uniform dress and nurse's cap when in clinic treating patients.[36]

## Community Outreach

The new curriculum created enhanced learning opportunities for students and allowed for additional oral health care to be provided in communities throughout Michigan. For more than 80 years, the school has been engaged in community outreach dentistry. In the late 1930s, help from the W.K. Kellogg Foundation enabled senior dental students to travel to county health departments in southwest Michigan to participate in one-week "field trips," as they were called at the time, to gain a better understanding of local oral health-care needs. In the 1950s, dental and dental hygiene students treated inmates at the Michigan State Prison in Jackson. Beginning in the late 1950s, dental students traveled to the Bay Cliff Health Camp northwest of Marquette during the summer to address

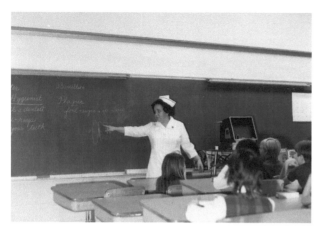

*Dental hygiene student, Melva Baxter, teaches dental health to elementary students during one of the early outreach experiences.*

the oral health needs of developmentally disabled children and adolescents ages 3–17. During the 1960s, dental hygiene students participated in summer fluoride programs throughout Michigan, applying topical fluorides to school-age children.

## Community Outreach Emerges

In the fall of 1971, the Department of Community Dentistry launched a pilot program for 3rd year dental students to visit various community health agencies to observe and verbally interact with members and patients at the agency. The pilot was so successful that the program was expanded to include 4th year students. No funds were allocated to support community outreach and all services were provided pro bono; yet the program grew and by 1974 participating agencies included Cassidy Lake Technical School, Milan Correctional Institution, Wayne County General Hospital, Washtenaw

Community College, Model Cities, Sumpter Health Center, and Saint Louis Boys School for the Retarded. The summer migrant program also added sites throughout the state. From the start, the students loved the opportunity to serve the community as well as to gain clinical experiences beyond the walls of the school. [37]

Outreach became so popular with the students that a lottery system had to be initiated to manage all of the students wanting to participate. Graduates generously gave back to the school with donations to support the program.

## Mobile Dental Vans

A research grant awarded to Dr. Robert Bagramian, chair of the Department of Community Dentistry with a PhD in oral epidemiology, allowed the school to purchase two fully equipped dental vans to use as mobile dental offices. The vans traveled among a group of select Ypsilanti and Willow Run schools. The five-year study was designed to determine the benefits of dental care given to school-age children. Dental care services included fillings, sealants, and fluoride and ultimately showed an 85-percent reduction in dental disease in the study population. When the study ended, Bagramian contacted the National Institutes of Health (NIH) and requested that the dental school be allowed to retain the dental vans. The NIH approved this request. Mobile dental units were exactly what the Department of Community Dentistry faculty needed to launch new outreach initiatives. The Community

Dentistry faculty ran this program until the vans were decommissioned in 1997.

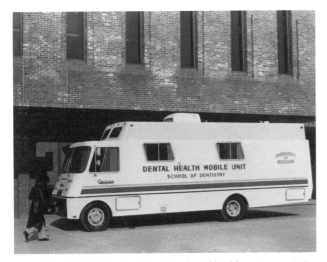

One of the School of Dentistry's mobile dental health unit vans sits in front of the building, ready for service.

"Initially, the concept of community outreach was not enthusiastically embraced by the clinical faculty. Since the outreach program was not a formal part of the curriculum, many faculty members were reluctant to give up control of clinical instruction in this way," Bagramian recalled when reflecting on the early years of the outreach program. But Bagramian persisted and after many meetings with the school's Executive Committee where he repeatedly made the case for community outreach experiences for students, he was given the green light to proceed. In the summer of 1972, the mobile dental units, each equipped with two dental chairs, dental instruments, and equipment that included an X-ray machine and sterilization facilities, traveled to a tomato-processing plant in Adrian,

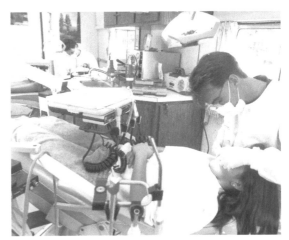

Jeffrey Daulton (DDS 1991, MS PedDent 1997) delivers dental care to a patient in the school's mobile dental unit. Anthony Bielke (DDS 1991) works at the dental chair in the rear.

Michigan, and provided dental care for the migrant workers at that site.

"Of course it didn't take long for the word to spread," Bagramian said. "The managers of a migrant site in Stockbridge heard about the dental services we were

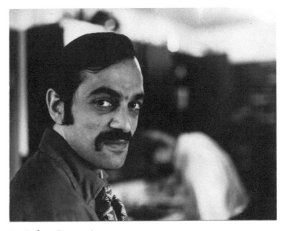

Dr. Robert Bagramian

providing in Adrian and said, 'How soon can you come to us.'"

Bagramian continued to champion the outreach program and the favorable results of the efforts in Adrian and Stockbridge led to the launch of the Summer Migrant Dental Clinic Program in the Traverse City area. The Traverse City program allowed 32 fourth-year dental students to spend two weeks each during the six-week summer program treating children and adults. About 3,000 migrant workers and their children received care. During the day, children between the ages of 4 and 13 received screening examinations, fluoride treatments, and other needed dental care. An evening clinic was set up so that the parents, who worked in the fields during the day, could also receive dental care. Another opportunity was made available to dental students to gain experience providing care to patients with special needs at a summer camp near Ortonville, just southeast of Grand Blanc, where they treated children with hemophilia.[38]

The outreach experiences have been highly regarded by dental students.

Students value the opportunity to care for patients they typically do not see in the School of Dentistry clinics. These experiences have also helped many dental students decide on a particular area of dentistry they enjoy or a specialty they wish to pursue. The success of the Summer Migrant Dental Clinic Program was a stepping-stone to a major expansion of the school's community outreach program in the spring of 2000.

## Community Dental Center

Community outreach took another step forward in January 1981 when the school, in cooperation with the city of Ann Arbor, established the Community Dental Center (CDC) at 406 N. Ashley Street in downtown Ann Arbor.[39] Once again, Bagramian saw an opportunity to provide special clinical experiences for the students, while at the same time providing much needed care to the underserved people of Ann Arbor.

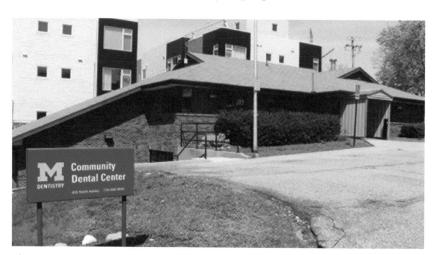

*The Community Dental Center in Ann Arbor.*

The clinic, originally housed in the Summit Medical Center, was setup as a component of Ann Arbor's Model Cities initiative that later was spliced into the federal Community

Development Block Grants (CDBG) program. The Summit clinic was woefully inadequate and a new dental clinic building was built at the north Ashley Street location with a $200,000 grant from the CDBG program. However, the dental clinic did not open as anticipated. When Bagramian learned of a vacant dental clinic in the heart of Ann Arbor, he immediately arranged a meeting with Mayor Louis Belcher. After listening to the ideas as to how the school could use the space and also help the community, Belcher said, "Get me a proposal as soon as you can."

The CDC was started by Bagramian (chair) and Paul Lang (faculty member) in the Department of Community Dentistry. It was, and still is, a joint cooperative venture between the City of Ann Arbor and the U-M. The city provided the building and limited financial support for the clinic, while the dental school provided equipment, staffing, and administration. The original goal for the CDC was that it be self-sustaining, providing a full range of oral health-care services for citizens of Ann Arbor and training for students in the area of dental public health, but subsequently it expanded its scope to include residents of Washtenaw County and clinical experiences for dental students.

Over the years, third- and fourth-year dental students have gained valuable clinical experience providing restorative, surgical, periodontal treatments, and emergency care. In recent years,

second-year dental students are there as well observing how a dental office runs, assisting the dentists, participating in infection control procedures, reviewing patients' health histories, and taking radiographs.

## Research

Since 1903, when Dr. Marcus L. Ward began to study the properties of dental amalgams used as a filling material, the School of Dentistry has been, and still is, recognized as a leader in dental research, both in basic sciences and clinical fields.[40] A lack of space in the 1908 dental building significantly limited research. With the addition of 21,000 square feet of laboratory space in the new Research Tower, there finally was room to accommodate the school's growing research enterprise.[41]

The School of Dentistry, in cooperation with the Medical School and the School of Public Health, requested the National Institute of Dental Research (NIDR) support the development of a university-based Dental Research Institute (DRI) on the Ann Arbor campus. In 1967, it was established. The purpose of the DRI was to formalize, expand, and better organize research training relevant to oral health. It was supported primarily by a grant from the NIDR of the U.S. Public Health Service.[42]

Michigan's DRI attracted leading scientists in microbiology, biochemistry, immunology pharmacology, physiology, and the emerging field of genetics. Clinical scientists in periodontology,

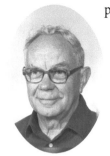

*First director of U-M's DRI, Dr. Dominic Dziewiatkowski, affectionately known as "Dr. J".*

pathology, and occlusion also joined this group. As a result, the DRI encouraged the development of multidisciplinary programs where basic and clinical scientists collaborated to address problems such as dental caries (cavities), periodontal disease, and others. Dr. Dominic Dziewiatkowski, recruited from The Rockefeller University, was named chair of the Department of Oral Biology and DRI director in July 1967. He served until 1972 and was succeeded by Dr. Harold Löe (1972–1975) and Dr. James Avery (1976–1989).[43]

The DRI was funded largely with federal grants. During the 1977–1978 academic year, sponsored research expenditures for the institute and the school totaled $2.42 million, with federal funds making up nearly $2.2 of that amount.[44]

## The Michigan Longitudinal Studies

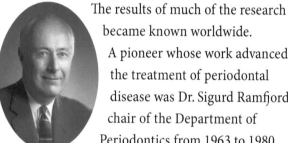

*Dr. Sigurd Ramfjord*

The results of much of the research became known worldwide. A pioneer whose work advanced the treatment of periodontal disease was Dr. Sigurd Ramfjord, chair of the Department of Periodontics from 1963 to 1980. Ramfjord and his team conducted the first longitudinal study of its kind in periodontics. For 10 years, they examined the effectiveness of four techniques used to treat periodontal defects: scaling and root planning (nonsurgical), gingivectomy (removing diseased tissue by surgery), flap surgery including osseous contouring, and the "Modified Widman Flap" which was not as invasive. Dr. Gloria Kerry (DDS 1956, MS Periodontics 1966) who worked in the Ramfjord lab said the results were extremely positive: "All the procedures were successful treatments when

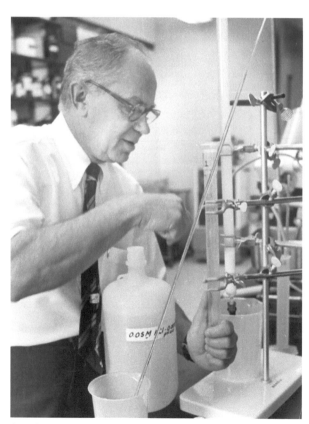

*"Dr. J." working in his lab.*

they were combined with visits for periodontal maintenance. . . . This meant that people could keep their teeth for many years and that old age didn't mean getting dentures."

## The Michigan Concept

Ramfjord organized the first world workshop on periodontics in 1966 where scientific goals for the field of periodontics were established. The results of his work led to the development of a dental education program that became known as "The Michigan Concept," a program that has been emulated worldwide.[45,46]

"This research made a lasting impact on future dental care," Kerry said. "Dr. Ramfjord should be remembered as a distinguished faculty member and as an inspirational mentor and teacher."

One dental student Ramfjord persuaded to return to Michigan to earn a master's degree was Dr. Gloria Kerry (DDS 1956).

"He urged me not to put off my studies and to come back to school and work for a master's degree in periodontics," she said. "But I had three small children; the youngest was three months old. I had to promise that I would complete my studies in three years and also complete my thesis." Kerry began working for her master's degree in periodontics in September 1963 and earned her degree in 1966.

Eight years later, Kerry said Ramfjord called her and asked if she would be interested in teaching periodontics at the School of Dentistry. Reluctant to do so because she was now raising five children, Kerry agreed to accept his invitation to start as an assistant professor.

Kerry said she enjoyed clinical dentistry in general and working with patients in particular. Ramfjord asked her to be a clinical investigator in a longitudinal study that was evaluating different methods of periodontal treatment. This revolutionary approach was Ramfjord's landmark study, the Michigan Longitudinal Studies, which began in the early 1960s. The statistically designed research included various periodontal treatments.

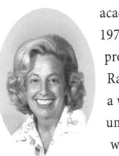

Dr. Gloria Kerry

Kerry successfully juggled both family and academic demands and in 1979, she was promoted to full professor with tenure. "To Dr. Ramfjord, I don't think having a woman in the program was unusual because women dentists were common in Europe. He treated me as an equal," she said.

## Student Table Clinics

In addition to research by faculty, dental and dental hygiene students and dental assistants were urged in the 1960s to participate in the school's "Table Clinics." These were tabletop demonstrations of techniques or procedures that focused on some phase of dental

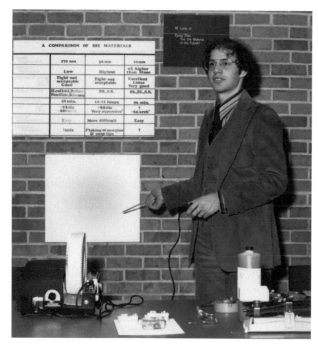

*The Student Forum was the site for the Table Clinic presentations.*

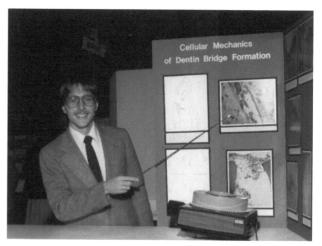

*Mark Fitzgerald presented his table clinic at the 1979 ADA national student table clinic competition. His table clinic won first place in the ADA competition.*

research, diagnosis, or treatment. Each student presented a 15-minute summary of their project which was often supplemented with visual aids, models, and casts.[47]

This was a competitive event and showcased student research. Some Table Clinic winners represented the School of Dentistry at the ADA annual session and competed with winners from other dental schools across the country.[48]

After the new School of Dentistry building opened in 1971, the table clinics were held on the ground floor in the Student Forum. As participation grew in later

years, the program was moved to the Michigan League Ballroom, where more space was available.

In 1979, Table Clinic Grand Prize winner Mark Fitzgerald represented the School of Dentistry during the ADA's annual session and won two major awards. One was as First Place winner in the ADA's national table clinic program and the Academy of Operative Dentistry's Outstanding Achievement Award. He was also invited to present his research at the annual meeting of the International Association for Dental Research and won second place in the Edward H. Hatton Awards competition for junior investigators. After earning his dental degree from U-M in 1980, he joined the School of Dentistry faculty as a part-time clinical instructor. He has been a full-time faculty member since 1990, holding the rank of associate professor

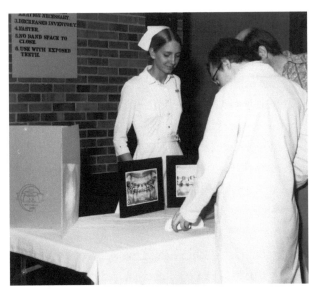

*Student participants in the Table Clinic program present a summary of their projects to faculty, staff, and students.*

and serving as associate chair in the Department of Cariology, Restorative Sciences and Endodontics. In 2017, Fitzgerald was named Associate Dean for Community-Based Collaborative Care and Education.[49]

The annual program, now known as Research Day, continues and is a forum that provides students a mechanism to showcase research projects they are involved in, share scientific interests with the dental school community, and develop professional communications as they present their research.

## We Write the Books

The school's reputation was continually enhanced as faculty members gained recognition for the textbooks they either published or edited. These texts were the ones commonly used in classroom and clinical education at dental schools nationally and internationally. This rich heritage is a source of pride for many U-M dentists and dental hygienists. One of the dental students and later a dental instructor was Dr. Jack Gobetti. "I had the privilege and honor of being educated by and teaching with some of the greats in dental education. Many of them, literally, wrote the books that we used in dental education. My professors were giants of our profession," he said.

Drs. Sigurd Ramfjord and Major Ash published *Occlusion* in 1966. According to the school's *Alumni Bulletin 1970*,[50] "the book is widely being used by dental schools throughout the world." The fourth edition was published in 1995. A prolific writer, Ash authored or coauthored other books that were published in French, German, Italian, Spanish, Portuguese, and Japanese.[51]

Other textbooks published by School of Dentistry faculty members that were widely used in dentistry included *Oral Diagnosis* by Drs. Donald A. Kerr, Major M. Ash, and H. Dean Millard (first published in 1959); *Differential Diagnosis* by Dr. Major Ash (1960); *Dental Materials: Properties and Manipulation* by Dr. Robert Craig (1975); *Oral Surgery* by Dr. James R. Hayward (1976); *Dental Materials and Their Selection* by Dr. William J. O'Brien (1978); and *Handbook of Orthodontics by D*r. Robert E. Moyers (1958, 1973).

In subsequent years, other School of Dentistry faculty members authored or coauthored important textbooks in dentistry and oral health. Some of those include *Basic Oral Physiology* by Robert M. Bradley (1981); *Oral Development and Histology* by Dr. James K. Avery (1994); *Essentials of Oral Physiology* by Robert M. Bradley (1995); *Essentials of Oral Histology and Embryology: A Clinical Approach* by Dr. James K. Avery and Professor Pauline Steele (2000); *Orthodontics and Dentofacial Orthopedics* by Dr. James McNamara (2001); *Treatment Planning in Dentistry* by Dr. Stephen Stefanac (2006); *Clinical Research in Oral Health* by Drs. William Giannobile and Brian Burt (2010); *Oral Health-Related Quality of Life* by Drs. Marita Rohr Inglehart and Robert Bagramian (2011); *Mineralized Tissues in Oral and Craniofacial Science: Biological Principles and Clinical Correlates* by Drs. Laurie McCauley and Martha Somerman (2012); *Osteology Guidelines for Oral & Maxillofacial Regeneration Clinical Research* by Drs. William Giannobile, Niklaus Lang, and Maurizio Tonetti (2014); and *Cone Beam Computed Tomography in Orthodontics: Indications, Insights and Innovations* by Dr. Sunil Kapila (2015).

## Reflections

A former faculty member who remembers Mann well was Dr. John Drach. Drach was interviewing for a faculty position in the Medical Chemistry program at the College of Pharmacy and at the School of Dentistry around the time the building was being constructed. Drach said he was not sure if he would get a teaching job at the School of Dentistry because he didn't have a dental degree. "I was a pharmacist and from my experiences working in drug stores, I realized dentists needed more education in pharmacology and therapeutics. Teaching those subjects to dental students seemed like a good idea," he said. Mann hired Drach to teach pharmacology, and U-M dental students benefited from his expertise from 1970 to 2007. During his tenure at the school, he chaired the Department of Oral Biology from 1985 to 1987 and chaired the Department of Biologic and Materials Sciences from 1987 to 2005.

"Dean Mann always had the interests of the dental school in mind. He was strict, but fair and true to his word. The school did well under his leadership," Drach said.

Mann retired on July 1, 1981, as dean of the School of Dentistry and director of the W.K. Kellogg Foundation Institute: Graduate and Postgraduate Dentistry. He served on the school's faculty for 41 years and as its dean for 19 years. The school's *Alumni News* noted in its fall edition, "His vision and administrative skills made possible far-reaching changes which resulted in the school being named first among dental schools in the country for its outstanding faculty, facilities and education."

*Chapter 2*

# The Doerr Years (1981–1982)

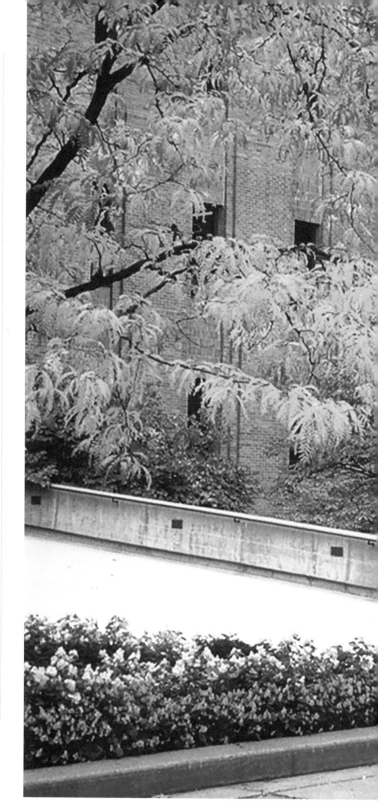

Dr. Robert E. Doerr was named interim dean by University of Michigan (U-M) Regents for a one-year term that began July 1, 1981, and ended July 1, 1982. As associate dean, Doerr worked closely with Mann and participated in much of the decision-making during the growth of the school in the late 1960s and early 1970s.[1] As Doerr stepped in as interim dean, the era of growth and expansion was waning and the school faced significant financial challenges and a decline in enrollments.

## A Surplus of Dentists?

The number of students receiving a DDS (doctor of dental surgery) degree from the School of Dentistry fluctuated between 100 in 1972 to as many as 151 in 1978.[2,3] Then, after all of the alarm expressed in the late 1960s over a projected shortage of dental health-care professionals, the tide suddenly changed and concern about a possible "oversupply" of dentists was being voiced during the late 1970s and early 1980s. However, fears of a surplus were not surprising.

During the 1971–1972 academic years, Mann wrote, "The enrollment and faculty will continue to expand for a few more years, but then a period of consolidation will take place. . . . The period of rapid growth in the student body and faculty will come to an end."[4]

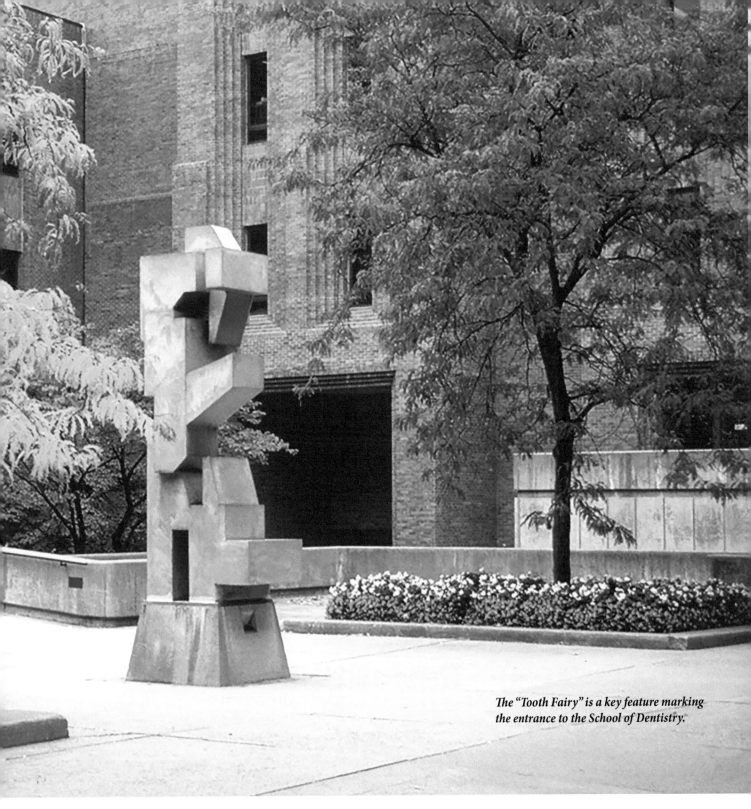

*The "Tooth Fairy" is a key feature marking the entrance to the School of Dentistry.*

## Budget Cuts

Advances in oral care, plus a recession in the late 1970s, an oil embargo, surging inflation, and a rise in unemployment, hit the national and Michigan economies hard. Budget reductions were inevitable and the School of Dentistry was significantly affected by these developments.

In a front-page letter that appeared in the spring 1982 issue of the school's *Alumni News*, Doerr wrote:

> Financial problems continue to plague the University and its schools and colleges. During the last three years the School of Dentistry has lost $750,000 from its general fund or base budget. We are now preparing plans for further reductions of one, three, and five percent for the 1982–83 year and a 10 percent reduction over the next five years.

## Enrollment and Tuition

The school requested permission from the state to lower enrollment to 125 students, a reduction of 25 per class or 100 over the four years of the dental program. Doerr noted that 100 fewer dental students would create a $375,000 shortfall in tuition revenue and that a tuition increase, perhaps substantial, would probably be needed during the next several years.[5] During the 1980–1981 academic year, tuition for a dental student was $3,168 for a Michigan resident and $6,060 for a nonresident. Four years later, tuition for a Michigan dental student was $5,256 and $9,940 for a nonresident during the 1984–1985 academic year.[6]

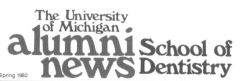

**The University of Michigan alumni news School of Dentistry**

Vol. 3, No. 2    Spring 1982

*It was a memorable weekend . . .*

### The 1981 Alumni Homecoming

"Fantastic success" describes the Fall 1981 School of Dentistry Alumni Homecoming.

Close to 500 alumni and their families returned to Ann Arbor November 6-7 and attended a weekend program of varied activities. Co-sponsored by the School of Dentistry Alumni Society and the Dental Hygienists' Alumnae Association, the event served both as a reunion for alumni and as a forum for discussion of current issues in periodontics.

Continuing education sessions all day Friday and Saturday morning addressed the topic "Trends in the Prevention and Treatment of Periodontal Disease." The scientific sessions were well attended and generated much discussion.

Luncheon in the Michigan League Ballroom on Friday featured a talk by Interim Dean Robert E. Doerr who shared with alumni his concerns and thoughts about problems facing the School and dentistry today. Prior to delightful entertainment by the U-M singing group The Friars, SDAS Board of Governors head Dr. William L. Shelton thanked all those who had a hand in making the Homecoming possible, par-

ticularly the Society's secretary Dr. J. Scott Fleming. Dr. Shelton also introduced Dean Designate Richard L. Christiansen who came from Washington, D.C., for the day's activities.

Holding special reunions that weekend were dental classes 1941, 1946, 1956, 1961, 1965, 1966, and 1971. Friday evening was a highlight time for the hygienists present, with a banquet at Weber's hosted by the Dental Hygienists' Alumnae Association.

Saturday dawned bright and clear, one of those perfect football afternoons in Ann Arbor that many will remember from their students days. In addition to education sessions in the morning, tours of the School and table clinics were enjoyed by alumni before adjourning to brunch at the League and then by charter bus to the stadium. An exciting football game with Illinois, which Michigan won 70-21 after trailing by 21 points in the first quarter, capped a wonderful weekend.

We urge you to start making plans NOW to attend the 1982 Homecoming, scheduled for the weekend of November 12-13, with Purdue as the football opponent. We guarantee an equally enjoyable time!

*Letter from the Dean*

Financial problems continue to plague the University and its schools and colleges. During the last three years the School of Dentistry has lost $750,000 from its general fund or base budget. We are now preparing plans for further reductions of one, three, and five percent for the 1982-83 year and a 10 percent reduction over the next five years. Your dollars have enabled us to replace some 13-year-old television equipment, upgrade the computer system, add to the student financial aid program, support 11 summer research fellowships for students, and provide travel for faculty to professional meetings. Thank you, again.

We are aware of the serious dental manpower problem, both within the state and nationally, and are working with the administration of the University, the governor's office, and the state legislature to achieve an initial reduction in the size of this fall's incoming class. Permission has been requested to limit enrollment to 125 students, a reduction of 25 per class or 100 over the four years of the dental program. In recognizing the manpower problem, the University has two primary concerns: one philosophical and the other practical. Philosophically, it is difficult to deny admission to highly qualified young men and women desirous of a career in dentistry. We have more than 700 applications this year and the purely educational argument is that we should continue at maximum enrollment when there are qualified applicants. In other words, a decrease in enrollment should reflect decreased demand for admission. The practical concern is that a decrease in enrollment of

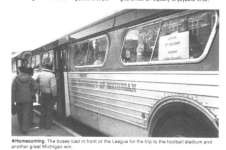

◆Homecoming. The buses load in front of the League for the trip to the football stadium and another great Michigan win.

(continued on page 2)

## Fund-raising Supplements Budget

To raise funds to meet potential shortfalls, the School of Dentistry named Dr. Richard Desmond to the newly created position of senior development officer in February 1981.[7] The need for additional funding sources was crucial. "In these days of financial cuts in state and federal sources of support, alumni aid is needed, both in contributing and in participating in fundraising events to help the school maintain its tradition of excellence," noted the school's *Alumni News* magazine in the summer of 1981.[8]

Desmond launched a series of phonathons that involved U-M dental students and alumni volunteer callers who spoke with 3,365 dental alumni about the school's recent achievements and some of the more pressing issues. In the fall of 1981, 12 phonathons were held and raised more than $164,000 from nearly 1,700 alumni. "Key to the success of the 1981 effort was the consistently enthusiastic participation of our alumni callers. They were every bit as effective as we knew they would be," he said.[9] By the time Desmond retired in 1990, he had been instrumental in increasing yearly gifts from $180,000 in 1980 to more than $1 million in 1988–1989 and 1989–1990.[10] Alumni support

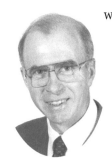

*Dr. Richard Desmond*

was tremendously important to the meeting the needs of the school providing greater sources of revenue, including endowments.

Succeeding Desmond was Richard Fetchiet. The early fundraising successes would set the stage for later school development initiatives that were part of the university's fundraising campaigns. Fetchiet and his team led successful campaigns in 1995 and 2009 and their efforts, on behalf of the school, continue today.

## Reflections

Doerr led the School of Dentistry as interim dean for a single year during a time when the school faced tough fiscal realities. He would not be deterred and the leadership he exhibited throughout his career in dentistry had more than prepared him to take on this formidable task. The population forecasts and the dental workforce survey he conducted had provided the data needed to convince the state legislature to fund the new building to meet the future dental workforce needs in Michigan. He then coordinated myriad details involved in the construction of the new building. He understood the dental school and its every operation better than anyone, and he worked tirelessly to see every task through to its successful completion. Throughout his career, he specialized in dental curriculum, evaluation, and individualized instruction and self-pacing for dental students. Doerr retired in 1986 following 35 years of distinguished service to the university.[11]

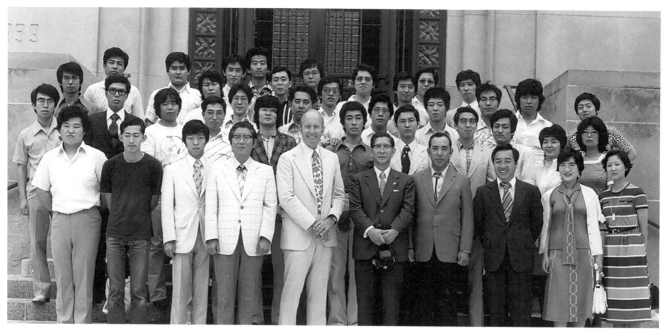

*Robert Doerr (front row, center) with the distinguished Japanese contingent from Masumoto Dental University.*

*Chapter 3*

# The Christiansen Years (1982–1987)

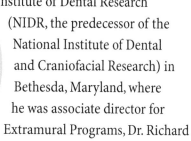

Arriving from the National Institute of Dental Research (NIDR, the predecessor of the National Institute of Dental and Craniofacial Research) in Bethesda, Maryland, where he was associate director for Extramural Programs, Dr. Richard Christiansen began his term as dean and director of the W.K. Kellogg Foundation Institute of Graduate and Postgraduate Dental Education on July 1, 1982. After his appointment was approved by University of Michigan (U-M) Regents at their June 18–19, 1980, meeting, U-M Vice President for Academic Affairs B.E. Frye said, "Dr. Christiansen has had a distinguished career in dental administration and research. His experience and abilities will serve our distinguished School of Dentistry well."[1]

## Budget Cuts Hit Hard

Christiansen faced financial challenges from the moment he arrived. "I knew about them when I accepted the dean's position in 1981," he said. "I spent

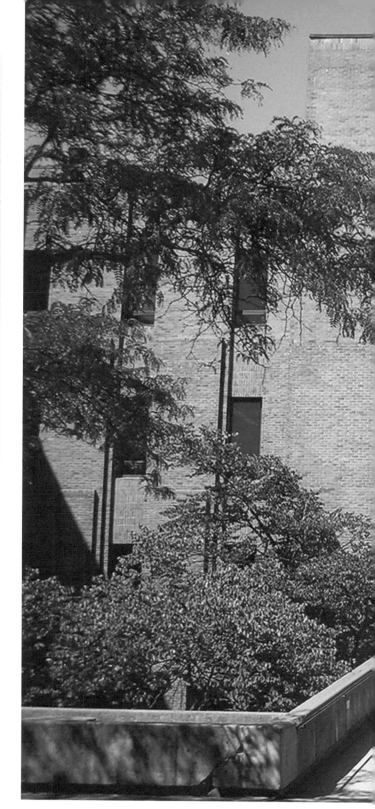

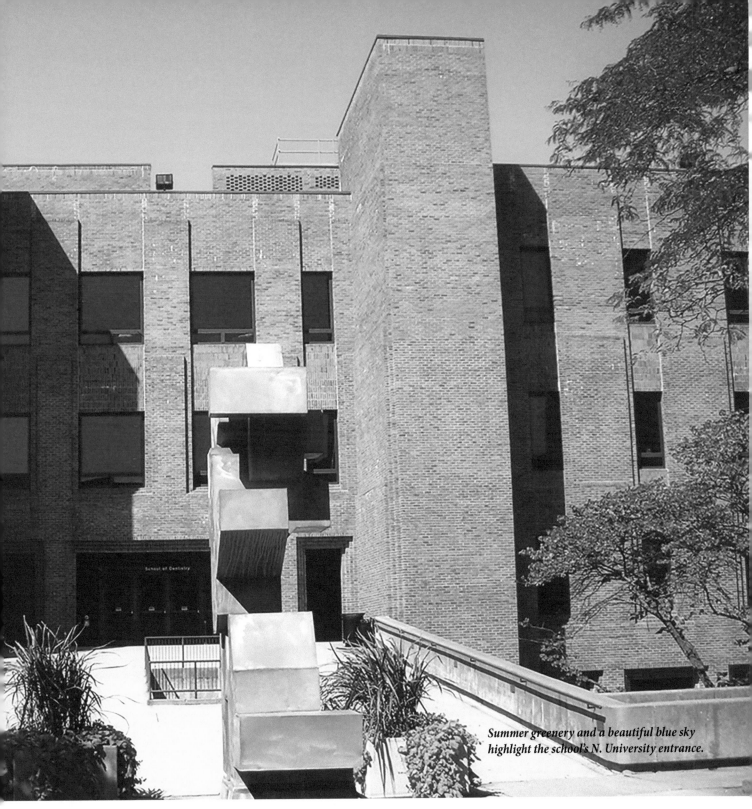

*Summer greenery and a beautiful blue sky highlight the school's N. University entrance.*

a lot of time conferring with Bob Doerr about finances and other matters."

In the 1981–1982 annual report from the school to the university, Christiansen noted: As with other units in the University, budget and financial matters occupied much administrative time, due to deteriorating economic conditions in the state. The school significantly reduced its 1981–1982 budget by $510,000 following a university mandate to make a 6-percent reduction. Vacant and unfilled positions were a carefully reviewed and not filling those positions contributed significantly to help balance the budget. No faculty positions were lost; however, the $510,000 reduction in spending was especially painful because many staff positions were cut. University statistics showed the school with 122 faculty members: 51 professors, 29 associate professors, and 42 assistant professors.[2]

## Managing the Budget Crisis

Christiansen appointed the school's Executive Committee to serve as a new Budget Priorities Committee to address budget shortfalls and make recommendations as to how to reduce school expenditures.[3] In a July 2, 1984, memo, Christiansen and Budget Priorities Committee Chairman Dr. Fred Burgett noted, "The crisis of the general fund shortfall exists and has to be dealt with. The fear of the Committee is that if the school does not contend with the deficit, the University administration will." He added that savings would include a headcount reduction of 16 percent of faculty and 23 percent in support staff. A July 19, 1984, follow-up memo noted: "The planned reduction is a viable one, the implementation of which will not detract from the educational, research and service missions of the school."[4]

For the 1983–1984 academic year, the school projected a general fund salary deficit in excess of $500,000, including fringe benefits. The following academic year was even worse with a General Fund deficit of $730,000. As a result, approximately 20 support positions were removed from the budget. Full-time equivalent (FTE) positions fell from 176.65 in September 1982 to 149.90 in 1984, a decrease of 15 percent.[3,5]

The number of FTE positions also continued to decline. By the fall of 1986, the school reported its FTE count for faculty was 134 and 143 for staff. The FTE reductions were more than 14 percent for faculty and more than 15 percent for staff.[6,7]

## Decreasing Class Size

Given the bleak budget picture, school administrators knew that it was imperative to reduce class size. For fall term 1982, 135 first-year dental students were admitted, a decline of 10 percent from the previous year. Future reductions were expected and by the start of the 1987 academic year, first-year dental student enrollment had declined by a third, from a peak of 151 students to 90 students.[8]

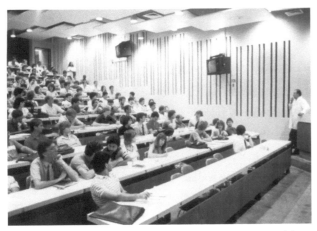

*Typical class listening to a lecture. In 1986, the class sizes ranged from 125 to 96.*

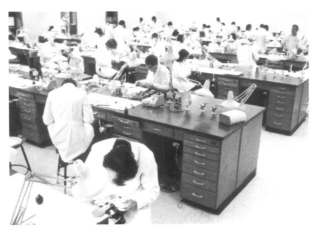

*First year DDS students working in the preclinical lab. The entering class size was 96 students in 1986.*

### DDS Enrollment 1981–1987

| Year | Applicants | Accepted | Enrolled | GPA | W (%) | Minority (%) | Out-State (%) |
|------|-----------|----------|----------|------|-------|--------------|---------------|
| 1981 | 873 | 173 | 150 | 3.39 | 28 | 11 | 3 |
| 1982 | 755 | 178 | 135 | 3.33 | 29 | 9 | 4 |
| 1983 | 666 | 183 | 125 | 3.29 | 26 | 14 | 6 |
| 1984 | 594 | 175 | 121 | 3.24 | 33 | 16 | 8 |
| 1985 | 503 | 175 | 121 | 3.26 | 36 | 15 | 15 |
| 1986 | 496 | 198 | 96 | 3.08 | 31 | 22 | 11 |
| 1987 | 566 | 201 | 90 | 3.11 | 39 | 28 | 16 |

*Source*: From School of Dentistry Transition Committee Report 1987, Section B: Introduction.

*Note*: GPA (Grade Point Average), W (Women)

## Engaging the Alumni

To help meet some of the budget shortfall, Christiansen also sought to establish endowed professorships that would also help the school recruit and retain highly qualified faculty. "There were clear signals that we wouldn't be able to rely on the same levels of state or federal funding in the future as we had in the past," he said.[9]

"I saw a need to get our alumni involved. I wanted the alums to be aware of the financial issues the school was facing and to enlist their help in supporting the school's programs," Christiansen said. "Dick Desmond in our Development and Alumni Relations Office worked closely with me to achieve those two important objectives." He underscored that that approach "was a good way to engage the alumni as we planned for the future and the related financial uncertainties."

## Browne and Najjar Endowments

In 1985, the school announced two major gifts from grateful alumni. Dr. Robert Browne (DDS 1952, MS 1959), a Grand Rapids orthodontist and chairman of the board and chief executive officer of Care Corporation, pledged $1 million to create an endowed professorship in dentistry. In making this gift, Browne noted:

> My contributions are a way of repaying the university for the opportunity it provided me. Alumni should want to see the high quality of the school maintained and even enhanced. . . . We all have a personal responsibility to help make that happen."[10]

Dr. Lyle Johnston was named the first Robert W. Browne Professor of Dentistry. Over the years, the Browne endowment grew to an amount that would support the establishment of a second professorship. In 2002, the Robert W. Browne Professorship in Orthodontics was established. Dr. Sunil Kapila was the first faculty member to hold this

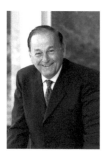

*Dr. Robert W. Browne*

professorship. See Appendix B for a complete list of the School of Dentistry endowed professors.

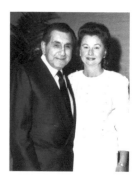

*Dr. William K. and Mrs. Mary Anne Najjar*

The school's second $1 million pledge was also designated to create an endowed professorship named for its donors, Dr. William K. and Mrs. Mary Anne Najjar.[10] After earning his dental degree from U-M in 1955, Dr. Najjar practiced dentistry in Grand Rapids for 14 years and started a dental materials company, Janar Corporation, which he later sold to Johnson & Johnson. Najjar said his reason for making this gift was based on his belief "in the future of the dental profession" and a desire to "reinvest some of my lifetime earnings in dentistry as a measure of my appreciation for the important part the University of Michigan played in my life." Dr. Martha Somerman was named the first William K. and Mary Anne Najjar Professor of Dentistry. As with the Browne endowment, the Najjar endowment also grew and was able to support a second professorship. In 2002, the William K. and Mary Anne Najjar Professorship in Periodontics was established and Dr. Laurie McCauley was the first faculty member named to this professorship.

## Dental Hygiene Programs Advance

Fall semester 1984, marked a milestone for dental hygiene education at Michigan with the launch of two new programs. A new baccalaureate degree program was introduced that included a one-year program of prescribed liberal arts courses followed by three years of didactic and clinical studies that included oral anatomy, radiography, dental pharmacology, pain control, nutrition, and other subjects. The change meant that all dental hygiene students enrolled in the College of Literature, Science and the Arts for their first year of study and completed years two through four at the School of Dentistry. A significant change was that students would no longer be accepted into the dental hygiene program directly from high school. Since this program was launched, all U-M dental hygiene students have graduated with a Bachelor of Science degree.[11]

The second program, a post-certificate program, was designed to provide dental hygienists who had graduated with an associate degree or certificate an opportunity to complete requirements toward a Bachelor of Science in dental hygiene. This program was offered for registered dental hygienists who either graduated from U-M or another accredited dental hygiene program.[5]

## Clinic Hours Expand, Clinic Managers Hired

Historically, departments staffed clinics in half-day sessions, with clinic instructors available either in the morning or afternoon. This arrangement posed a great challenge to students trying to provide comprehensive care or complete oral health care to patients coming to the school's clinics for treatment. A significant change to the clinical program began in May 1986 when the school's clinical departments established all-day clinics. This meant that students could consult with faculty instructors in specific disciplines in every clinic session.

In the summer of 1985, four clinical managers were hired to supervise and instruct fourth-year dental students. The clinic manager's job was to help students learn practice management skills and manage their patient's treatment more effectively. The managers also assisted in assigning patients to students. Since this program was well received by students, faculty, and patients, Christiansen

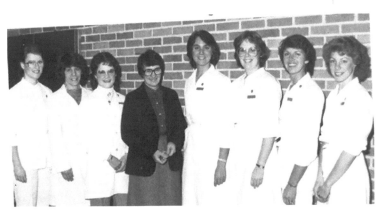

*1984 dental hygiene faculty: (L–R) Jennifer Turnbull, Wendy Kerschbaum, Debra Zahn-Simmons, Sally Holden, Tamara Bloch, Bridget Clancy, Susan Pritzel, and Susan Johnstal. From 1984 School of Dentistry Student Yearbook.*

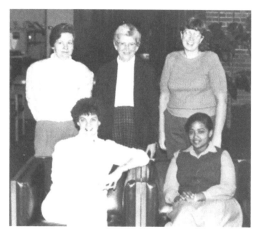

*The new clinic managers were highlighted in the 1987 Student Yearbook. Seated: Bridget Kilpatrick and Wanda Winborn. Standing: Paulette Haibel, Della Sell, and Marsha Meyer.*

expressed a desire to add more managers for dental students in the second and third years of their education.[6,7]

## Hospital Dentistry and Oral Surgery Move

Another important change in clinical care came on February 14, 1986, when the Department of Hospital Dentistry and the Department of Oral and Maxillofacial Surgery moved from facilities in the old University Hospital to the new U-M Hospital. The new space offered 10 examination/treatment rooms, 2 equipped for ambulatory oral surgery, and a fully equipped recovery room. With new administrative, patient care, and patient waiting areas, the space was two-and-a-half times larger than that in the old outpatient building.[12,13]

## The Dental Research Institute

Christiansen had a keen sense of the research environment in dentistry. Having served as associate director for extramural programs at NIDR and director of the organization's craniofacial anomalies program before coming to Michigan, he was aware of trends taking place nationally. He had a good idea of how these trends might affect dental education.

One important trend involved a decline in oral disease, primarily dental caries. That trend suggested the way oral care was provided to patients would have to change. Christiansen emphasized that dentists in the future would need to become more broadly educated in all facets of oral health in order to provide optimal care. "Future practitioners," he said, "must have an education that emphasizes a thorough understanding of scientific principles, human biology and basic biologic sciences in addition to the rigorous clinical disciplines."[14]

After his years at the National Institutes of Health (NIH), Christiansen also recognized the importance of the NIH-funded Dental Research Institute (DRI) on the U-M campus. He was well versed in how DRIs functioned at U-M and four other locations around the country.

"One of my goals was to foster and promote the advancement of the most promising areas of dental/oral-facial research, which was vital for leadership in the profession of dentistry," he said. During the 1984–1985 academic year, it seemed that funding the DRIs was in jeopardy as Congress began to consider budget reductions for these institutes. Christiansen testified before the House Budget Committee to defend the NIH-funded DRIs. He spoke about their importance to oral health care nationwide. The funding cuts did not occur.

## The Michigan Growth Study

Also in 1986, Dr. James McNamara, who began teaching in the Department of Orthodontics during 1983–1984 academic year, was asked by Dr. Fred More, associate dean of the School of Dentistry, to assume a new role as curator of the university's Elementary and Secondary School Growth Study.

The Michigan Growth Study, as it was later known, began in 1935 in the University School, a laboratory within the School of Education. Over time, the study became world famous with data collected and used in hundreds of research studies. Launched by Dr. Willard Olsen, dean of the School of Education, dental records, radiographs (X-rays), and dental casts of young children and teenagers were updated annually from 1935 to 1970. The data gave oral health-care professionals a wealth of information about how and to what degree the growth and development of a child's craniofacial structure occurred. Information also included medical, physiological, and anthropologic data. Only 9 or 10 schools in North America collected such longitudinal data.

The collection was brought to the School of Dentistry in 1952 when Dr. Robert Moyers became chair of the Department of Orthodontics. "The information is a valuable resource and continues to be used in clinical studies to this day because it serves as a benchmark or reference point to help us know how children without treatment grow and develop," said McNamara. Moyers also was the founding director of another initiative that McNamara became extensively involved with, the Center for Human Growth and Development. Established by U-M Regents in 1964, the center recruited senior scholars (fellows) from many disciplines who developed interdisciplinary and collaborative research programs integrating craniofacial biology, developmental psychology, developmental biology, nutrition and public health, morphometrics, anthropology, and pediatrics.[15]

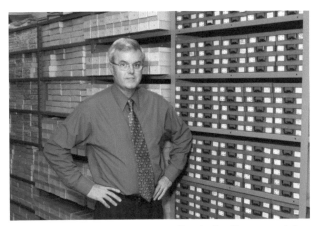

*Dr. James McNamara stands in front of hundreds of boxes containing research study models.*

## Technology and Learning

The school's 1986–1987 annual report to the university noted the academic year had been an exceptionally busy period for the television unit. The basic activities of the videotape production team, which included a total of 92 productions that year, along with videotape duplication, audio/visual services, and maintenance, continued to absorb a major portion of the staff's time. The school underscored its commitment to the growth of computers in the academic environment. A completely renovated computer center, CAIDENT (Computer-Aided Instruction DENTistry), opened on October 17, 1986, included 34 Macintosh computers, 13 dot matrix printers, a laser printer, and a generous assortment of software. The school recognized that the computer would continue to play an important role in student learning and the production of educational materials.[7]

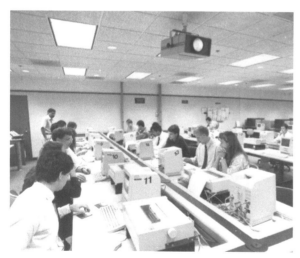

*Students use the CAIDENT center computers to access course materials available to them electronically.*

## Nurturing International Collaborations

The School of Dentistry was recognized as a leader in dental education and research around the world. The school's faculty understood the value of international collaborations and began to work on several international exchanges with dental schools and dental organizations.

When he was at NIDR, Christiansen traveled to Jerusalem in 1979 to help the Hadassah School of Dental Medicine celebrate its 25th anniversary. That experience had an impact on him that remained with him during his years as dean. "I thought that if we could get professionals from around the world together to discuss oral health needs on a global scale it might lead to tackling issues and solving problems more efficiently and effectively," he said.

In May 1984, Christiansen, joined by Edith Morrison (assistant professor in Periodontics) and U-M alums Joseph Cabot (DDS 1945) and Hugh Cooper Jr. (DDS 1951), participated in a visit to the Peoples Republic of China. The trip was sponsored by the American Dental Association at the special request of the Chinese Medical Association (CMA). The CMA asked members of the 17-person delegation to consult with its professionals on programs that included dental education, public health, research, and organized dentistry. The visit paved the way for future connections between U-M and a number of schools throughout China.[16]

Student exchanges with Nippon Dental University in Japan were established in 1986. That same year, the school and the University of Berne School of Dental Medicine in Switzerland signed a sistership agreement. A signing ceremony took place in the Washington, DC, at the home of the Swiss ambassador.[17]

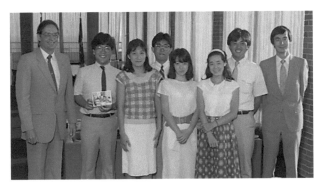

*Student visitors from Nippon Dental University pose for a photo with Dean Christiansen in the Faculty Alumni Lounge.*

## Reflections

In a memo to the dental school faculty, Christiansen announced on March 18, 1987, that he would not seek a second five-year term as dean. Reflecting on his five years as dean, Christiansen said:

> It was an exciting time, not just here at the school, but in the profession too. I have no doubt I made the right decision to come to Michigan. The dental profession was changing, and I wanted to be a part of that change and help shape the new direction dentistry was taking, both academically and clinically.[18]

During his tenure as dean, Christiansen initiated relationships with nine foreign schools of oral health. He was involved in the establishment of the International Union of Schools of Oral Health in 1985. In the late 1980's he served as a Project Hope consultant in Krakow, Poland. He reviewed the Krakow dental school and helped design, plan and complete the Project Hope Hospital. This was done before Poland became liberated from the Soviet Union. In June 2000, he was awarded an honorary doctorate degree from Nippon Dental University, Tokyo, Japan.

Christiansen's commitment to global outreach didn't end when he stepped down as dean. In 2015, a generous gift from Christiansen and his wife, Nancy, established the Richard Christiansen Collegiate Professorship in Oral and Craniofacial Global Initiatives. Dr. Carlos González-Cabezas, director of the school's Global Initiatives in Oral and Craniofacial Health program was named the first Christiansen Collegiate Professor. The Global Initiatives Program extends the Christiansen legacy as it strives to improve global oral health and promote health equity through education, research and patient care. Dr. Richard Christiansen retired from U-M in January 2001. He holds the titles of Dean Emeritus and Professor Emeritus.

*Chapter 4*

# The Kotowicz Years (1987–1989)

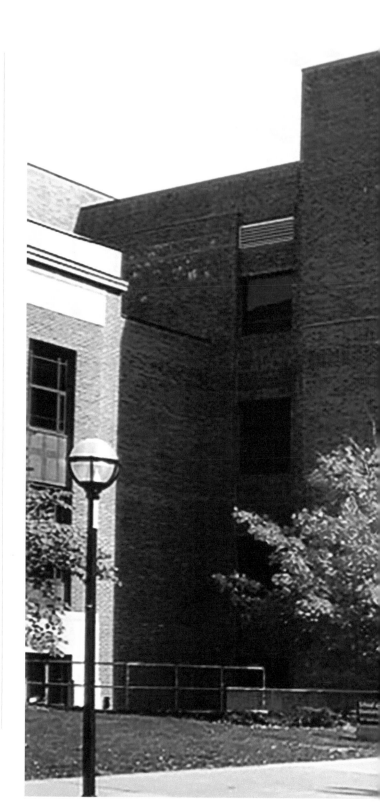

Nine days after Dean Dr. Richard Christiansen announced that he would be stepping down as dean, University of Michigan (U-M) Provost James Duderstadt visited the school to meet with the faculty and express his appreciation to Christiansen for his efforts to reposition the school in a very rapidly changing environment. Some of those changes included managing a declining enrollment, an oversupply of dentists, a shift in how dentistry was being practiced, and the rise of new technologies.

## The Transition Committee

Duderstadt also announced that he had named Dr. William Kotowicz as interim dean. As interim dean, Kotowicz had been asked to chair a Transition Committee. This committee would work closely with the provost to chart the future course of the school. Duderstadt emphasized that during this time of transition, the school needed to assess its strengths and weaknesses, develop a vision for its future, cut the number of departments, revise its curriculum, and find ways to become more integrated with the rest of the campus. "The school continues to be somewhat isolated from the rest of the campus in general and the other health science disciplines in particular," Duderstadt said.

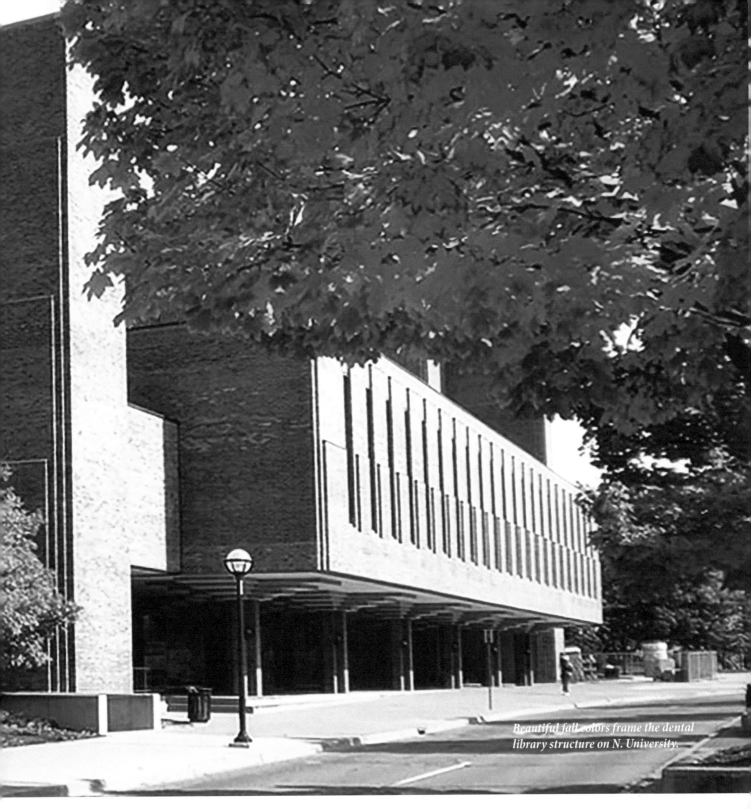

*Beautiful fall colors frame the dental library structure on N. University.*

Christian Stohler, who was then the chair of the Department of Occlusion, says he recalls the Duderstadt presentation very well:

> I remember when James Duderstadt came to the dental school to tell everyone during an assembly, in no uncertain terms, that change would take place at the dental school. That, I think, was *the major* turning point for the school. . . . More importantly, once changes began to occur, the dental school became a truly important part of the University of Michigan. Previously, the school wasn't in sync with the university. Duderstadt made it clear that the dental school and its faculty members had to interface with and participate in broader university activities. And they did. (Personal communication, March 10, 2015)

Duderstadt also stressed the need for quick, effective action.

> Time is short. Externally, the health care environment is changing very rapidly, and other professions and institutions are responding. If the University of Michigan is to retain its leadership position in dentistry, we must move forward quickly and courageously. We do not have the luxury of lengthy planning or an extended search for new leadership.

> Challenges bring risks. . . . When we depart from well-established pathways, both the journey and the destination become less predictable. I press you for this major planning effort now. . . [and] I am confident of your ability and commitment to work together to bring about a future that will expand the rich heritage of the School of Dentistry.[1]

## Interim Dean

On July 1, 1987, Kotowicz became interim dean and head of the Transition Committee. Duderstadt said he named Kotowicz to both positions "because he enjoys an unusual degree of respect and support across broad segments of the school. His recent service as a member of the school's Executive Committee provides both an appropriate perspective and important credibility for this important role." Duderstadt concluded by "asking you as faculty to give full and strong support to Professor Kotowicz and the Transition Committee as they work with you to achieve change and restore the school to a position of true national leadership."[1]

Duderstadt, who was named president of the U-M in 1988, later reflected on that appointment:

> In the mid-1980s, when the School of Dentistry was facing a serious crisis, the faculty pointed to Bill Kotowicz as the person they would respect and trust most with the leadership of the school. This trust has been well founded, since Bill has provided strong, fair and wise leadership of the school through and since those difficult times.[2]

## A Common Purpose and Hard Work

The Transition Committee led by Kotowicz included faculty members Kenneth McClatchey, Charlotte Mistretta, Raymond Fonseca, Joseph Regezi, and John Lillie. The members of the committee came from both inside and outside the dental school and gelled as a team to tackle this daunting yet critically important task. The committee was charged with the task of taking a top-to-bottom look at all dental school operations and creating strategies to address the challenges it faced.[3]

The first charge the committee had to address was to streamline the organizational structure and function of the school by reducing the number of departments. Confronting the issue head on, 18 departments were consolidated into 6. Reducing the number of departments "put Bill Kotowicz in a difficult position because it was tough to tell some faculty members that they were no longer department chairs," said Dr. John Drach. "Bill did his best not to alienate the older more established faculty members because they were experts in their field and essential to the school."

Pending faculty approval, the new departments were named as were interim chairs. The new departments were the following: (1) Prosthodontics (Brien Lang), (2) Restorative Dentistry—included endodontics, occlusion, and periodontics (Joseph Dennison), (3) Biologic and Materials Sciences (John Drach), (4) Oral Medicine, Pathology and Surgery (Raymond Fonseca), (5) Prevention and Health Care Delivery—included and dental hygiene (Robert Bagramian), and (6) Orthodontics and Pediatric Dentistry (James McNamara).[4]

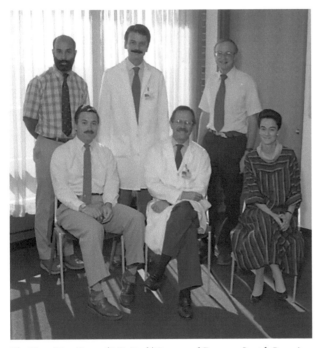

*The Transition Team: (L-R, Back) Raymond Fonseca, Joseph Regezi, John Lillie. (L-R, Seated) Kenneth McClatchey, William Kotowicz and Charlotte Mistretta.*

**Dr. Charlotte Mistretta**, a member of the Transition Committee, remembers the countless early morning meetings members of the Transition Committee attended to address their charge. The members met regularly for three hours on Monday mornings for over a year and frequently at additional times.

Reflecting back on the work of the committee, Mistretta recalls:

> We were given a formidable task and a relatively short timeline to get the job done. Our backgrounds and academic and professional focuses were varied but remarkably, we gelled and worked extremely well together. We set to task and a year after our initial meeting we presented our plans for administrative and department restructuring, curriculum revisions, faculty appointments and promotions, a full set of Bylaws, budgeting and financial planning and research operations to a distinguished external advisory committee.

These external experts included Howard Bailit, senior vice president with Aetna Health Plans, George Keller, senior vice president with Barton-Gillet Company and Bernard Machen, associate dean at the University of North Carolina. The external advisory committee was impressed with the plans

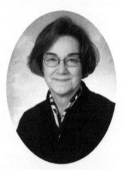

*Dr. Charlotte Mistretta*

they reviewed and lauded our efforts to reconfigure the administrative structure and redesign the curricular strategies to insure the school would regain its academic posture within the university, revitalize its research enterprise and employ a sustainable budget model moving forward.

The feedback from the external advisory committee validated all of the hours of hard work and thoughtful deliberation the committee members invested in the transition process. The Transition Committee could succeed because we had an uncommon, outstanding leader and "person for the times" in Bill Kotowicz, and the full backing from the University's Central Administration in our decisions. (Personal communication, May 25, 2017)

## Administrative Reorganization

Consolidating the department structure meant each department was responsible for more areas of study within the department. Administrative operations and decision making were decentralized, giving the departments tremendous authority to develop their internal organizational structure, budgets, research, faculty development, and fundraising. "This environment supports mentoring and career development and enhances our ability to recruit high-quality faculty. In addition, evidence of that success is validated by how frequently our administrators and faculty members are recruited by other dental schools, often to be deans," Kotowicz said.[5]

The school also rethought how academic and other administrative units would collaborate and share resources. The Transition Committee organized administrative duties according to function: admissions, student affairs, curricular matters, graduate and postgraduate education, clinical and hospital affairs, computer operations, continuing education, and research. Kotowicz said that research would become a high priority at the school and that faculty would be expected to invest more time and resources in research.[4]

Another important objective tackled during the transition process was to amend the school's faculty appointment policies and bring them in line with university-wide promotion and tenure procedures. A later addition of the "clinical track" further addressed

## Musings on Major Changes

Dr. Christian Stohler joined the U-M School of Dentistry as an associate professor in 1984 and chaired the Department of Biologic and Materials Sciences from 1996 until 2003, when he was named dean of the University of Maryland dental school. Since 2013, Stohler has been dean of Columbia University's College of Dental Medicine.

In a March 10, 2015 personal communication Stohler said:

> [The Transition Committee] helped everyone focus on what needed to be done. But committee members had a horrible job. They had to develop a new leadership structure that made a lot of people unhappy, especially reducing the number of departments from 18 to six. But there was no way a person could manage a school with so many departments. The school had to develop a structure that was more efficient and led to more accountability.

*Dr. Christian Stohler*

Stohler himself was directly affected:

> I was one of those who was no longer a department chair. I remember submitting my resignation as chair of the Department of Occlusion on a Friday afternoon and the following Monday morning I was part of another department (Restorative Dentistry).

The school's transformation was not a one-, two- or three-year event. Stohler said:

> It took about 10 or 11 years to accomplish. . . . It was very hard work. It was painful. But it was a major achievement that was very important to the school and the university. The Transition Committee tried to create something visionary that would help both the school and the university well into the future. Bill Kotowicz, as head of the Transition Committee, and other committee members did a remarkable job.

Dr. Jed Jacobson concurs:

> The reorganization, or the transition, the school experienced was one of the most difficult, yet meaningful events I witnessed when I was at the school. I think it made everyone realize that,

> we as a school, had to bring value to the University of Michigan and become an integral part of the fabric of the university. (Personal communication, July 23, 2015)

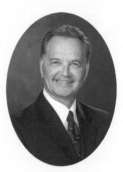

*Dr. Jed Jacobson*

the teaching needs of the school as well as provided an advancement series for the clinical faculty. (Personal communication, September 18, 2017)

## A New Curriculum Emerges

When the Transition Committee was evaluating the school's infrastructure and programs in 1987, it expressed concern that the predoctoral curriculum had not changed substantially in 20 years. A seven-member Curriculum Task Force (CTF) was convened to take on the task of reviewing and revising the DDS curriculum.[6]

The CTF, made up of representatives from each of the six new departments, took a multi-tiered approach, assessing the strengths and weaknesses of the existing curriculum, setting guidelines to develop a new program of study, then designing the new curriculum, and determining how best to implement it. The CTF proposed that the time scheduled to deliver this curriculum be increased from 4,500 hours to 4,700 with more time available to the students for the mastery of clinical skills. They also stressed that the number of hours the students were in contact with the curriculum be held at 32 each week. To achieve this goal and provide more time for clinical instruction, the CTF suggested the following: (1) extending the academic year, (2) reducing redundancies in didactic clinical material facilitated by the consolidation of departments, and (3) integrating and resequencing the basic science curriculum.

Dr. John Lillie—chair of the Curriculum Task Force, associate professor of dentistry, and professor of anatomy and cell biology—explained the changes in the September 12, 1988, issue of *The University Record.* "Most of the traditional curricula were based on specialties of dentistry," he said. "We've tried to integrate those disciplines and build toward a new concept of comprehensive treatment planning and patient care."

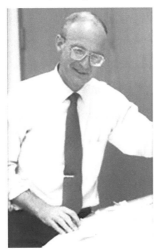

*Dr. John Lillie led the curriculum task force that designed the new curriculum.*

*A drafting table was used to map out the complexities of the new curriculum.*

## Members of the Curriculum Committee Task Force

Previous department affiliation noted in parentheses.

Chair of the task force:

**John Lillie, DDS, MS, PhD**—Anatomy & Cell Biology, Medical School, Oral Medicine/Pathology/Surgery (Oral Surgery)

Members of the task force:

**Sharon Brooks, DDS, MS**—Oral Medicine/Pathology/Surgery (Oral Diagnosis & Radiology)

**Fred Burgett, DDS, MS**—Restorative Dentistry (Periodontics)

**Richard Fisher, DDS, MS**—Prosthodontics (Periodontics)

**Ron Heys, DDS MS**—Restorative Dentistry (Operative Dentistry)

**Dennis Lopatin, DDS, PhD**—Biologic and Materials Sciences (Oral Biology/Immunology)

**Frederick More, DDS, MS**—Orthodontics & Pediatric Dentistry (Pediatric Dentistry) and also associate dean for Predoctoral Academic Programs and Student Affairs

## Goals of the New Curriculum

The new predoctoral curriculum embraced four main goals and the school's faculty and staff were resolute in their commitment to realize each of them. Earlier clinical experiences, year-round classes and clinics, and the initiation of a new comprehensive patient care program emphasized the development of patient care and practice management skills.[7]

| *Goals of the New Curriculum* |
|---|
| Goal 1: Build an intellectual foundation for each student in the basic and applied sciences |
| Goal 2: Develop the skills necessary to provide comprehensive dental care |
| Goal 3: Foster an understanding of the impact of dental health and health-care behavior on decisions made by governmental, insurance, and commercial groups on health-care issues |
| Goal 4: Instill a commitment to continuing professional development after graduation through participation in profession organizations, community activities, continuing education, and attention to current literature in the field |

*Source*: Excerpt from the Curriculum Plan submitted to the Transition Committee.

Each year from 1988 to 1991, segments of the new curriculum were submitted to the full-time faculty for review and approval. Then, as each new segment was finished, students and faculty provided feedback on course structure and how the course fit with those around it. Data from these evaluations helped identify content overlap or gaps and were useful to make adjustments before the course was offered next. By the fall of 1991, the new curriculum was fully implemented and patient-centered comprehensive care became a focal point of every dental student's clinical experience.[8]

## Student Research Flourishes

The U-M School of Dentistry has a long-standing history of engaging students at all levels in research activities through both externally funded formal research training programs and participation in faculty research projects.

At the predoctoral level, the students benefited from a training grant entitled "Short-term training in health professional schools" funded by the National Institute for Dental Research (NIDR). The grant supported approximately 12–15 students per year and that number was generally matched by the School of Dentistry.

Together these funding sources supported as many as 30 Student Research Program participants each year. The student projects were presented at the annual Table Clinic program, later to become Research Day. Many of these student projects were submitted to and accepted for presentation at the annual International and American Associations for Dental Research (IADR/AADR) meetings.

In 1987, the AADR created a student research fellowship program in an effort to encourage and support predoctoral student research in U.S. dental schools. School of Dentistry students were encouraged to apply for these fellowships and some applications were funded. As a member of the School of Dentistry's Fellowship Review Committee, Biologic and Materials Sciences faculty member Dr. Dennis Lopatin observed that the successful applicants were generally the individuals who had worked on a project for a year, were conversant in the scientific literature related to their project, and worked closely with their faculty mentors during the application preparation process. As a result, the applications were very strong and successful. (Personal communication, May 19, 2017)

Lopatin and the Review Committee set a policy whereby all Student Research Program participants who wished to participate in the program for a second year were required to apply for an AADR Student Research Fellowship. The U-M student applicants became so successful in obtaining AADR fellowships that after several years, when Michigan student scientists were awarded the lion's share of the fellowships, AADR instituted a rule that limited the number of fellowships awarded to any one school.

In 1988, Lopatin and Jed Jacobson assumed responsibility for the management of the Student Research Program which until then was run primarily during the summer break of about two and a half months. With the implementation of the new curriculum, the summer break was now shortened to six weeks and staggered by class year. This seriously impacted the Student Research Program and jeopardized NIDR support due to fewer weeks available for students to actually complete a research project.

Lopatin, principal investigator on an NIDR short-term training grant and other faculty colleagues, developed a plan that integrated aspects of the 10-week summer student research program into the DDS curriculum. Now, throughout the academic year, students worked with their mentors to develop their research protocols and attend seminars on various aspects of research. The continuous, ongoing research experience, combined with an intense lab or clinic-based experience during the summer break, satisfied the NIDR requirements for research exposure and the grant renewal was approved.

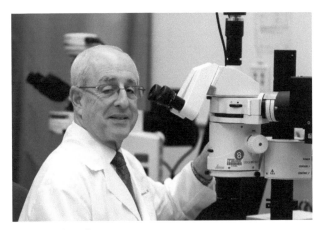

*Dr. Dennis Lopatin*

## U-M—OSU Research Duel

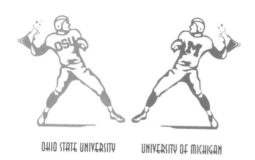

OHIO STATE UNIVERSITY    UNIVERSITY OF MICHIGAN

In 1987, Walter Loesche, professor and director of research, created what was called the UM–OSU Research Duel. The duel, coordinated by Biologic and Materials Sciences faculty member Dennis Lopatin and Samuel Rosen at The Ohio State University (OSU) Dental School, was a Table Clinic competition held annually between

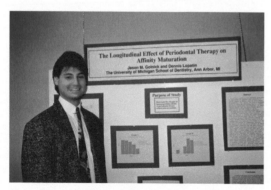

*Jason Golnick (DDS 1994, MS PedDent 2003) with his U-M/ OSU Research Duel poster.*

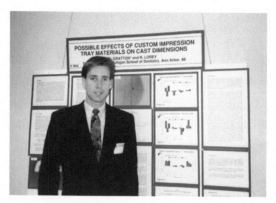

*David Gratton (DDS 1994) with his U-M /OSU Research Duel poster.*

predoctoral students of both schools. The host school alternated from year to year, one year in Ann Arbor and the next year in Columbus. [9]

Students from each school's student research program were selected to present their research in a "friendly" competition, judged by faculty members from both schools. Of interest, one of the OSU judges was a junior faculty member, Dr. Laurie McCauley, who in 2013 would be named dean of the U-M School of Dentistry. While there was a "traveling" plaque recording the winner of each duel, the true benefit of the duel was the experience the students gained in discussing their research with other faculty and students and getting a glimpse of what learning dentistry was like at the host school.

## Preparing for the Future

To prepare dental students for the challenges of the 1990s and beyond, Kotowicz often emphasized to students, faculty, and alumni that dentistry was on a new path. It was evolving from a primarily technical profession ("drill and fill") to one that combined advances in dentistry, medicine, biology, and other areas of science; and that it was vital for U-M dental students to be prepared. The new curriculum was designed to educate highly competent practitioners in an environment that mirrored a general dental practice.

In line with that thinking and realizing the importance of collaboration with other schools and colleges, Kotowicz reached out to utilize the resources available throughout the rest of the U-M. This included collaboration with the School of Public Health, the

College of Pharmacy, and the College of Engineering. More involvement with the Medical School was also initiated in areas that included geriatrics and oncology.[7]

The dental hygiene program also experienced changes during this time. Professor Pauline Steele retired in 1988 after 20 years of service and was succeeded by Professor Wendy Kerschbaum. Kerschbaum was the third director of the dental hygiene program since its launch and held that position until 2012, when she was succeeded by Professor Janet Kinney.

## Recruiting Faculty

A drive to increase the number of faculty members to teach both academic dentistry and clinical dentistry was a high priority. In the early 1970s, most faculty members were part-time instructors and had their own private practice. Finding qualified young faculty members to teach at the School of Dentistry was difficult. In many instances, dental practitioners had built their practices and were hesitant to leave for salary levels that were lower in academia than in private practice.[10]

In 1972, the school's faculty totaled 239 (both part time and full time). Included in that number were 71 clinical instructors, 50 assistant professors, 49 professors, 25 clinical assistant professors, 23 associate professors, 7 instructors, 7 lecturers, 4 visiting assistant professors, and 3 clinical professors. Not included

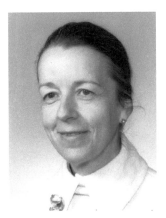
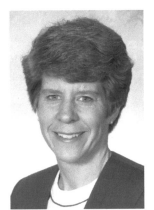

*Professor Pauline Steele*     *Professor Wendy Kerschbaum*

in those numbers were 20 Medical School faculty members who also taught at the dental school.[11]

Faculty recruitment efforts began in earnest in 1988 with searches in periodontics, operative dentistry, prosthodontics, biologic and materials sciences, and occlusion. Kotowicz said the positions would not be easy to fill and that candidates "must be superior teachers with strong research potential."[7]

## Reflections

The school, guided by the Transition Committee and the efforts of various task force groups, proceeded with initiatives essential to the future success of the dental school. The departmental and administrative structures were reorganized. The dental school bylaws were written and executed, the promotion and tenure document was created, curricular changes were implemented, comprehensive care was introduced, and the budget was balanced. Kotowicz was confident that a new dean "would be named or in place" by the fall of 1989 and felt that these initiatives would "provide an excellent base for a permanent dean."[7]

On June 29, 1989, U-M Provost Charles Vest came to the Kellogg Auditorium to announce that J. Bernard Machen, associate dean of the School of Dentistry at the University of North Carolina—Chapel Hill, would become the new dean of the U-M School of Dentistry on October 1. Vest also praised Kotowicz: "Bill has risen to this occasion and has just performed, I believe, an outstanding service to this school, the university and the profession."[12]

*Chapter 5*

# The Machen Years (1989–1995)

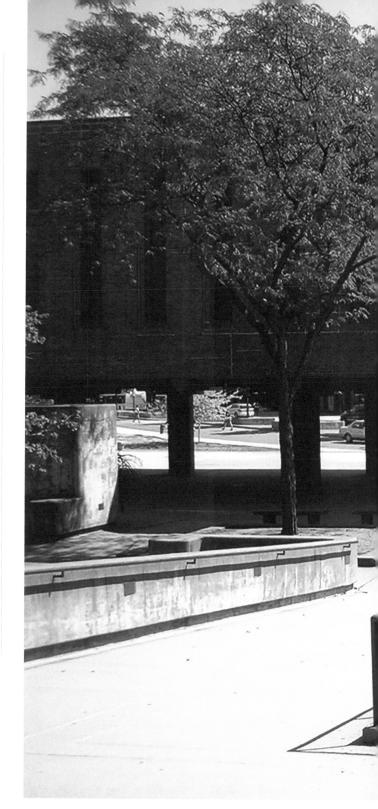

About nine months before J. Bernard Machen arrived at the School of Dentistry to begin his term as dean, Dr. John Drach said he was asked by Interim Provost Robert Holbrook to chair the Search Committee and recommend three candidates to the provost. The committee, Drach said, was looking for several attributes in a new dean—a dentist with academic credentials beyond the DDS plus organizational, managerial, and financial experience. From a list of over 50 candidates, the Search Committee ultimately recommended three names, including Machen's, to the new provost, Charles Vest, and James Duderstadt, who was now president of the University of Michigan.

Machen started his tenure as dean on October 1, 1989. "It was no secret that the School of Dentistry was going through some very difficult times when I came to Michigan in 1989. Alumni and others knew it. The school was downsizing, there were budget issues and other concerns," Machen said reflecting on the realities of the academic climate in the late 1980s.

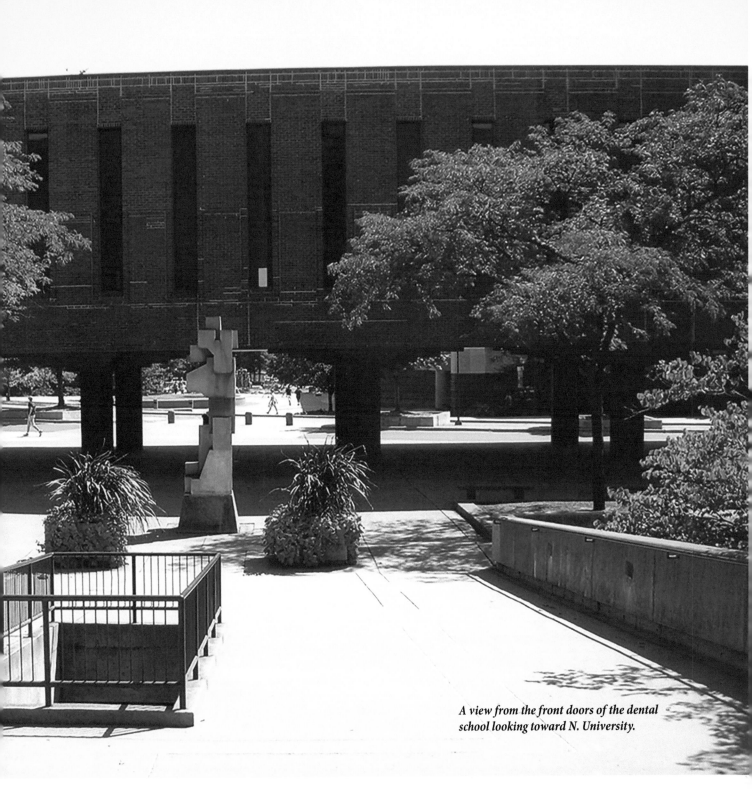

*A view from the front doors of the dental school looking toward N. University.*

## Maintaining the Momentum

As he started his deanship, Machen said it was "absolutely essential we continue the activities started during the past two years."[1] In addition to the many initiatives advanced by the school during the transition period, he spoke of the necessity of continually improving the school's educational and clinical programs. He stressed the need to develop new interdisciplinary research activities that cut across departmental and school boundaries as well as the importance of developing graduate education programs that contributed to the needs of society in the twenty-first century.

In his first address to faculty on October 23, 1989, Machen referred to the goals and principles that were identified by the Transition Committee in 1987. But he went a step further saying,

> I am formally endorsing this thoughtfully drawn list of goals and taking it as my own. . . . By endorsing these goals, I hope to make it clear that I want to continue in the direction that has been identified during the transition process."[2]

To sustain the momentum established by the Transition Committee, Machen also announced that he was appointing Kotowicz as senior associate dean. "In my mind, this is the most important appointment I will make at the school," he said, adding Kotowicz "will be an integral part of the administrative team. This appointment has enthusiastic support from within the dental school and from the general university."[3]

## New Organizational Structure

After some tweaking, the new department structure was finally set in place on July 1, 1990, when the school's Executive Committee voted to approve the major realignment of the school's six departments.

**School of Dentistry
Department Configuration**

- Biologic and Materials Sciences (which included biomaterials and oral biology)

- Cariology and General Dentistry (which included endodontics, occlusion, operative dentistry, and practice management)

- Oral Medicine, Pathology and Surgery (which included hospital dentistry, oral and maxillofacial surgery, oral diagnosis, and oral pathology)

- Orthodontics and Pediatric Dentistry (no change in content or focus)

- Periodontics, Prevention and Geriatrics (which included community dentistry, dental hygiene, and periodontics)

- Prosthodontics (which included complete denture prosthodontics, fixed partial denture prosthodontics, and removable partial denture prosthodontics)

*Source: Alumni News Supplement,* March 1990, p. 1.

During this time, the Office of Patient Services was created to support the delivery of quality dental care and ensure that clinic operations ran smoothly and efficiently. Dennis Turner, who directed the preclinical dentistry program was named director of the new office in 1991 and a year later was named assistant dean for patient services. In these capacities he implemented the integrated preclinical science program, the patient/student monitoring system, and the new D-3 clinical program. He also directed the implementation of the vertical integrated clinical program in the predoctoral education program and was instrumental in the redesign and implementation of a new central sterilization system and a centralized record program.[4]

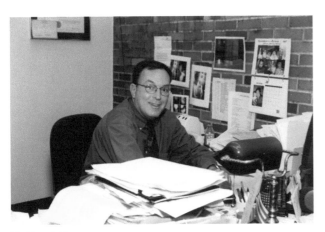

*Dr. Dennis Turner*

A Patient Records office was also established to track each patient's dental record and to efficiently process the services completed at each appointment. Managing patient records in this way introduced a new level of accountability, linking each record to a specific provider thus significantly reducing the likelihood of a "kept, lost or missing" chart.[5]

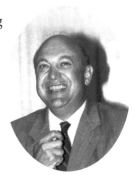

*Dr. Arnold Morawa*

Administrative restructuring also included the formation of a new unit in 1990, the Office of Alumni Relations and Continuing Dental Education. The new unit combined the areas of continuing education, an initiative that began in 1933 [6] with alumni relations, development, and publications. Dr. Arnold Morawa was named the assistant dean of the new office and was tasked with coordinating the activities of the unit with the goal to enhance connections and communications with the school's alumni.[7]

## Phasing in the New Curriculum

An emphasis on comprehensive care changed the focus of clinical care provided by dental students. Service to the patient became the priority, so that a patient was no longer viewed as a means to fulfilling a set of requirements for graduation, but as an individual whose specific dental needs would be addressed through a comprehensive treatment plan.

In 1990, a pilot program was initiated in one of the D4 clinics that offered fourth-year dental students the opportunity to apply comprehensive care practices to patients they were treating. The program was a success and the following year, the pilot program was expanded to include all *three* clinics where fourth-year dental students provided care.[8]

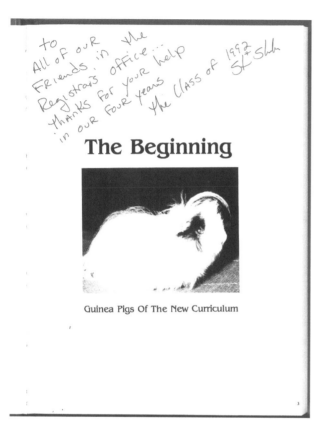

## The Beginning

Guinea Pigs Of The New Curriculum

*This page from the 1992 dental school yearbook captures the sentiment of the students who were introduced to the new curriculum.*

In each of the three clinics, a generalist/master clinician was named clinic director to oversee the team approach to diagnosis, treatment planning, patient care, and maintenance. The clinic directors were assisted by specialists in prosthodontics, endodontics, and periodontics on a continual

basis with oral surgeons, orthodontists, and oral pathologists available as needed. This interface among the generalist, specialist, and student created a supportive environment conducive to cooperation, planning, and education.

One of the major goals of the third-year curriculum was to increase the D3s clinic time in preparation for comprehensive care in the D4 year. By increasing the length of the school year and by eliminating the duplication of didactic material, an additional 122 hours of clinical experience were incorporated into the D3 year.

To manage this increase in clinical services, a computerized system was developed to track patients from recall and preventive services through planned restorative services. The system was designed to maintain a patient pool for the school and assure continuous comprehensive care service for patients.

## Building a Strong Faculty

With the new department structure in place, Machen named the chairs who would lead those departments. John Drach was named chair of the Department of Biologic and Materials Sciences. He was interim chair of the Department of Oral Biology since 1985 before it became a part of the Department of Biologic and Materials Sciences. Joseph Dennison was named chair of the Department of Cariology and General Dentistry, and Brien Lang was name chair of the Department of Prosthodontics.

Following extensive national searches, three other department chairs were named. Lysle E. Johnston, Jr.,

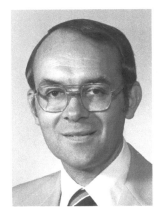

Dr. John Drach

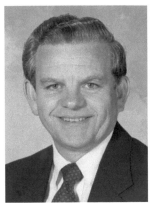

Dr. Joseph Dennison

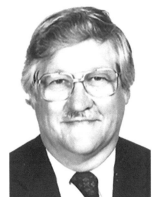

Dr. Brien Lang

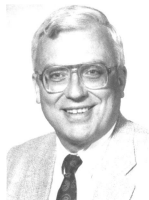

Dr. Lysle Johnston

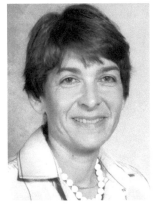

Dr. Martha Somerman

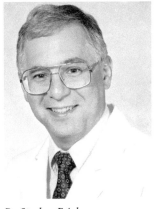

Dr. Stephen Feinberg

was selected to head the Department of Orthodontics and Pediatric Dentistry. He was also appointed the Robert W. Browne endowed professor, named for the Grand Rapids orthodontist who established one of the school's first faculty endowments in 1985. His appointment as department chair and director of the Graduate Orthodontics Program in 1991 was tantamount to a homecoming since he earned his dental degree and master's degree in orthodontics from the U-M in 1961 and 1964, respectively.[9] He was a renowned expert in the differential effects of various orthodontic treatments and mechanisms of facial growth and the nature of interactions between growth and treatment. He taught more than 300 orthodontic specialists during his

career, lectured worldwide, and received some of the most prestigious awards in orthodontics before he retired in May 2005.[10]

Martha Somerman came to the School of Dentistry as chair of the Department of Periodontics, Prevention and Geriatrics. She was the first woman to chair one of the school's academic departments. Internationally recognized for her work with mineralized tissue proteins, her research on tissue regeneration and repair would become the basis for innovative research and possible new clinical therapies involving bone implants and tissue repair.[11] She was also the first to hold a professorship, endowed in 1985, by one of the school's alumni, Dr. William K. Najjar (DDS 1955) and his wife, Mary Anne.

On September 1, 1990, Dr. Stephen Feinberg began his tenure as chair of the Department of Oral Medicine, Pathology and Surgery. He came to U-M from the Ohio State University College of Dentistry, where he had taught since 1983. In making the appointment, Machen noted the high praise Feinberg received as an effective teacher. Feinberg's basic laboratory research focused on tissue regeneration and his clinical work examined temporomandibular joint surgery.

**Dr. Martha Somerman** said Machen tried several times to get her to come to Michigan.

> I told him I wasn't interested, but he was persistent. I was lucky he kept trying, because looking back, my experiences at the U-M School of Dentistry played *an indispensable role* that significantly allowed me to expand my expertise far beyond dentistry and science to a much larger skill set, one that included recruiting excellent faculty, staff and students; better understanding of shaping communications messages; different or new approaches to education; and expanding what I knew about critical basic science investigations and their potential translational applications.

When hiring new faculty, Somerman said:

> [She didn't hire them] just to be the drivers of research in mineralized

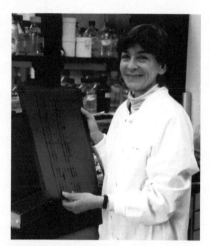

*Dr. Martha Somerman in her lab.*

> tissues. I was interested in faculty who were innovative thinkers with a collaborative spirit and who embraced what an academic environment offered – an opportunity to connect with students in the classroom and collaborate within the school and on a larger scale, be it at the university level, nationally and internationally. (Personal Communication, April 21, 2015)

## New Technology Advances Dental Education

New technology, which included desktop computers, modems, and use of the Internet, were now being used with increasing frequency in education and patient care.

In 1991, Joseph Dennison, chair of the Department of Restorative Dentistry, and Machen discussed creating a one-year program for recently graduated dentists who planned to practice comprehensive general dentistry and who also wanted to expand their skills in areas of personal interest. An Advanced Education in General Dentistry (AEGD) program was established following those discussions. The program offered didactic instruction and

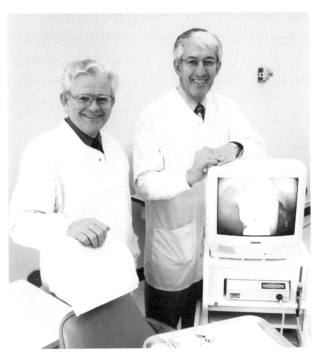

*Drs. Joseph Dennison and Peter Yaman demonstrate the Veravision UltraCam II Intraoral Camera System.*

clinical experiences in all specialty disciplines in dentistry. AEGD emphasized esthetic dentistry and use of esthetic dental materials and techniques, practice management, and geriatric dentistry and included internal rotations in oral surgery and pediatric dentistry.[12]

Using technology to help patients was also the focus of a course in advanced esthetic dentistry techniques for fourth-year dental students. Developed by Restorative Dentistry faculty members Dennis Fasbinder and Donald Heys, the course provided didactic and laboratory instruction on the use of computer-aided design and computer-aided manufacturing (CAD/CAM) technology that students were then able to incorporate in treatment plans for appropriate cases in clinic.[13]

Helping launch the AEGD program on July 1, 1992 was its new director Dennis Fasbinder, who was beginning his teaching career at the School of Dentistry.[14]

Three U-M dental graduates enrolled. Technology was an important part of the AEGD curriculum. "I was fortunate to get in on the ground floor of the technology initiative here and the launch of AEGD," Fasbinder said. As technology continued to evolve during the 1990s, CAD/CAM became accepted and incorporated into the AEGD curriculum.

"AEGD gave recent dental graduates new insights into ways they could provide better oral health care to their patients using emerging CAD/CAM technology," he said. The CEREC (Chairside Economical Restoration of Esthetic Ceramics, or CEramic REConstruction)

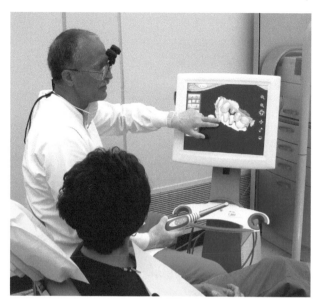

*Dr. Dennis Fasbinder uses computer-aided design and computer-aided manufacturing (CAD/CAM) technology to describe treatment options to a patient.*

system by Sirona enabled dentists to fabricate and insert ceramic restorations into a patient's mouth at chairside during a single visit instead of requiring multiple visits.

Fasbinder was director of the AEGD program until 2013, when it was replaced by a new program, Computerized Dentistry. Computerized dental systems are an integral part of contemporary dental practice. The new program was designed to provide students a focused opportunity to apply dental technology as part of comprehensive patient care.

In 1993, an official from Nobel Biocare's headquarters in Sweden visited the school to discuss a new high-tech approach to make titanium all-ceramic crowns—the Procera® System. Company

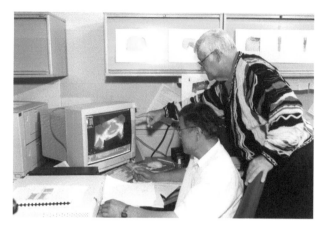

*Dr. Brien Lang (R) and Rui-Feng Wang review a computer generated image of a Procera® bridge.*

representatives were interested in collaborating with the school to investigate clinical questions related to dental implants and all ceramic crowns—questions critical to patient care. The collaboration, led by Brien Lang, chair of the Department of Prosthodontics, resulted in a $625,000 gift from Nobel Biocare and the establishment of a Center for Excellence.

Over the next five years, the center conducted more than 50 research projects and became the research hub

The Procera® scanner was able to measure more than **60,000 separate points** on a die in minutes with extreme precision. In seconds, data collected during the scan was sent by modem to Stockholm. A few days later, a patient's crown or bridge was delivered to the School of Dentistry for placement.[15]

for answering laboratory questions and conducting clinical evaluations on implants and restorative devices. The technology involved was innovative and according to Lang had "the potential to revolutionize dentistry." The center set a benchmark for excellence in teaching, research, product evaluation, and patient care.

## National Conference on Workforce Diversity

Diversity was always emphasized as essential to the school, the university and the oral health profession. In June 1991, more than 170 health professionals from around the nation gathered at the University of Michigan for a conference, Black Dentistry in the 21st Century. Hosted by the School of Dentistry, and co-chaired by Drs. Michael Razzoog and Emerson Robinson, the meeting featured discussions about dental

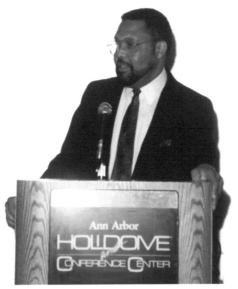

*Dr. Emerson Robinson welcomes the participants to the Black Dentistry in the 21st Conference.*

care in the Black community, the state of dental practice in the Black community, health behavior and research.

Conference participants voiced concern about a shortage of minorities in the health profession. One of them, guest speaker Dr. Audrey Manley, deputy assistant secretary for health in the Department of Health and Human Services, noted that Blacks accounted for 12% of the U.S. population, but only 4% of the nation's dentists and 5% of the nation's physicians. "Minority America is sorely in need of practicing dentists, physicians, researchers, academicians and scientists who are sensitive to cultural and ethnic distinctions, and who can serve as mentors and role models for our youth," she said.[16]

Recommendations that emerged from the conference included:

- Recruitment initiatives to familiarize students about dentistry in the high schools and through counselors, dental school faculty, dental practitioners and professional organizations.

- Extend outreach programs into high schools and colleges to encourage early exposure to involvement in research.

- Remove barriers to preventive practice by insisting on inclusion of preventive procedures in all health plans that provide dental benefits.

- Establish a level of responsibility within the African-American community to oversee funding and research efforts.

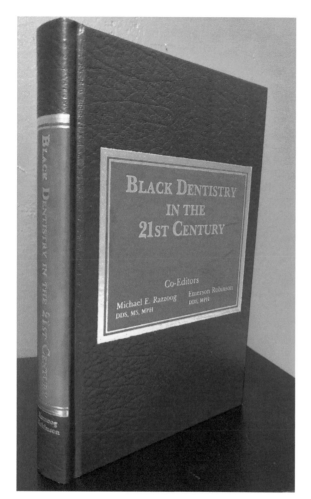

*The proceedings from the 1991 national conference on black dentistry in the 21st century.*

- Create a data bank of African-Americans interested in faculty and administrative positions and a network to monitor institutional commitment. [16]

Proceedings from the conference were later published in a book, *Black Dentistry in the 21st Century*, co-edited by Drs. Razzoog and Robinson.

## Machen Reappointed

In September 1993, Machen was reappointed as dean through 1999. Without a doubt, significant progress on all School of Dentistry fronts had been made. Speaking to the faculty and staff on September 23, 1993, Machen thanked everyone for their hard work. He said the school's financial outlook had improved, research support continued to grow, the number of applications for admission to both the dental and dental hygiene programs was growing, and master's programs and residencies had strong applicant pools. "I can state with confidence that today the University of Michigan School of Dentistry is among the leaders and best," he said. [17]

"The direction of our school is now under *our* (his emphasis) control," he said. "To be successful in the twenty-first century, it will be necessary to continue to make significant changes." His priorities moving forward included developing a new program to educate dentists in the clinical specialty education programs, creating a high-quality PhD education program in the oral health sciences (OHS), and taking a new look at the academic dental hygiene program. "These four programs – dental, master's, PhD and dental hygiene – are the academic core of our institution," he said. [17]

## Research in the 1990s

Collaboration was the operative word in research during the 1990s. In his October 1989 address to faculty, Machen said developing new interdisciplinary research activities that cut across departmental and school boundaries was among his highest priorities.

An OHS/PhD program began taking shape in the early 1990s. The school's sole PhD program was in oral biology. Machen asked Dr. Charlotte Mistretta to launch a school-wide doctoral program, drawing on the talents of faculty members from all six departments.[18] The expanded OHS/PhD program, directed by Mistretta, was officially established in 1994.[19] The OHS/PhD program was needed because, as then senior associate dean, William Kotowicz said,

> …dental education and dental research needed well-educated PhD-level researchers. Since the PhD is the ultimate academic degree, we knew that if we wanted to remain competitive and continue attracting both the best faculty and the best students, we would have to have a school-wide program and build it, literally, from the ground up.[20]

## The Campaign for Michigan

Under the umbrella of the University's billion dollar Campaign for Michigan, publicly launched in 1992, the School set a goal to raise $10 million for student support, faculty support and facility renovation projects. Because alumni and friends were so generous and the early response to the school's effort was so positive, the initial $10 million goal was increased to $13 million. The grand total at the end of the campaign was nearly $29 million, boosted by a $10 million dollar gift commitment from Dr. Roy Roberts (DDS 1932) and his wife, Natalie. At the time, the gift from the Roberts was believed to be the largest single commitment ever made to a dental school.[21]

## The Sindecuse Museum

In 1990, Dr. Gordon Sindecuse (DDS 1921) suggested to Dean Machen that the school create a dental museum that would collect, preserve, and exhibit memorabilia showcasing dentistry's growth and evolution. To make that happen, Sindecuse gifted $1 million to establish what would become the Gordon H. Sindecuse Museum of Dentistry.[22] The museum officially opened on September 18, 1992, under the direction of curator Jane Becker.[23]

Becker's first tasks were to acquire a basic collection, create storage for the artifacts, and coordinate the installation of exhibits. The initial exhibits were crafted from the collections of three dentist collectors. Charles C. Kelsey (DDS 1964), a prime keeper of the school's history, had assembled a chronological exhibit of dental articulators. Ronald D. Berris (DDS 1974) lent items from his personal collection including a "Swan" dental chair (ca. 1870), an X-ray unit (ca. 1930), early Ritter electrical dental unit (ca. 1920), and an array of dentifrice containers with advertising images underglazed on the porcelain lids. Ohio dentist Jack Gottschalk, knowing that items would be well cared for and kept together, allowed the museum to purchase artifacts from his private collection. The first exhibits recreated two operatories from two distinct historical periods—an operatory setup from the late nineteenth century before electricity was common and an early electric operatory when electricity was used primarily for lighting and running water.

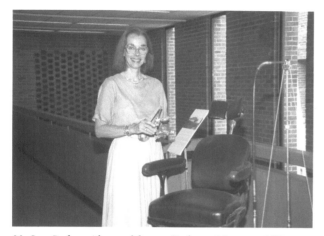

*Ms. Jane Becker with one of the new Sindecuse Museum exhibits.*

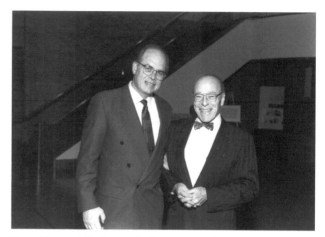

*Dean J. Bernard Machen with Thomas M. Graber.*

Sindecuse's gift made it possible to purchase collections, renovate the W.K. Kellogg lobbies, and establish an endowment to ensure perpetual support.[23] His gift to establish the museum, however, would not be his last. By 1995, outright gifts from Sindecuse, coupled with his estate gift to the school, exceeded $4 million.[24]

## Another Endowed Professorship

A new endowed professorship was established in April 1995. World-renowned orthodontics researcher and clinician Dr. Thomas Graber formalized a $1.2-million commitment to the School of Dentistry to fund the Thomas M. Graber Professorship in Orthodontics.[25]

Graber, an orthodontist and anatomist, had a major impact on the treatment of craniofacial anomalies in dentistry and medicine. He had served as a visiting faculty member in the Department of Orthodontics since 1958 and said, when making this gift, that

"despite the fact that I'm affiliated with the University of Illinois, I consider Michigan's Department of Orthodontics to be the best in the country." Dr. James McNamara was appointed as the first Thomas M. and Doris Graber Endowed Professor.

## Machen Appointed Provost

After successfully leading the school through major changes and two years into Machen's second five-year term as dean, U-M President James Duderstadt asked Machen to serve as the university's interim provost and executive vice president for Academic Affairs. On June 20, 1995, Machen announced that he would move from the School of Dentistry to the Fleming Building to become interim provost.

> I want to emphasize that this is a *temporary* position. I am not a candidate for Provost, and I expect to resume my deanship of the School of Dentistry as soon as a replacement has been

named. . . . Senior Associate Dean Bill Kotowicz, an immensely competent administrator, will be serving as acting dean in my absence – as he did before my appointment.[26]

Machen served as interim provost for a year, then, with the resignation of U-M President James Duderstadt, the Board of Regents asked Machen to extend his term for two years (1996 and 1997) and assume the role Provost and Vice President for Academic Affairs. Machen agreed to take on the provost's responsibilities under one condition: that he be allowed to name his successor at the dental school. William Kotowicz, who was senior associate dean at the time, then was named interim dean in the fall of 1995.

## Reflections

The transition and subsequent department reorganization along with the implementation of the new curriculum were among the hallmarks of the Machen years. Drs. Jed Jacobson and Lisa Tedesco offered poignant insight into Machen's tenure as dean,

Dr. Jed Jacobson said:

> Looking back at that period of time, I believe Bill Kotowicz and the work of the Transition Committee he led played a major role in the success Bernie had as dean at the School of Dentistry. . . . The transition or reorganization of the dental school worked. The school went from being a very independent unit on campus to one that was woven into the fabric of the university.

The University of Michigan brand with prospective dental students became a powerful one. As a result of the school's achievements since then, we have been one of the pre-eminent dental schools in the world. (Personal communication, July 23, 2015)

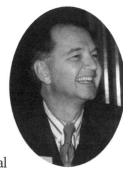

*Dr. Jed Jacobsen*

Dr. Lisa Tedesco, who joined the School of Dentistry in July 1992 as associate dean for Academic Affairs and as a professor in the Department of Periodontics, Prevention and Geriatrics, lauded Machen's and Kotowicz's leadership:

> Both played major roles in making change materialize at the school. They were change agents and what they did was absolutely essential. Bernie and Bill understood higher education and its valuable role in society. They understood Michigan's responsibilities, the resources that were needed to create and maintain faculty support, and the importance of diversity in society. (Personal communication, June 8, 2015)

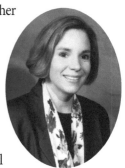

*Dr. Lisa Tedesco*

Machen left the U-M to become the president of the University of Utah from 1998 until 2004, when he was named president of the University of Florida—a position he held through December 2014.

*Chapter 6*

# The Kotowicz Years (1995–2003)

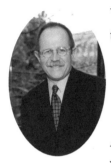

With Dr. J. Bernard Machen's temporary assignment and new responsibilities in the Fleming building, Bill Kotowicz, once tapped for special service, was this time appointed as interim dean. As senior associate dean, Kotowicz was closely connected to all of the programs and initiatives going on in the school. He was in an excellent position to advance the mission and goals of the school.

## Competition for Spots

The school continued to experience growth in the size and quality of its first-year applicant pool. Competition among prospective first-year dental students became more intense. The number of applications submitted to the school by prospective dental students was on the rise and by 1997 totaled 1,621 (i.e., 16.2 applications for each of the 100 places in the class).

## The New Model for Clinical Education

A key component of the new curriculum proposed by the Transition Committee and the Curriculum Task Force was the emphasis on clinical education for students and comprehensive, patient-centered oral health care for patients. The objectives of this holistic approach were to make dental education more effective and efficient as well as to improve patient care.[1]

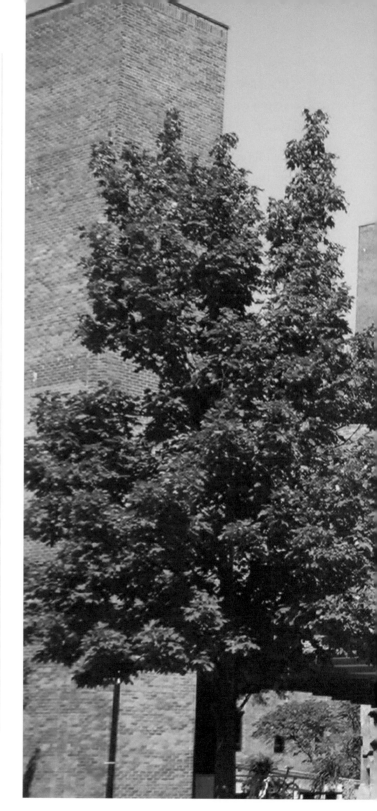

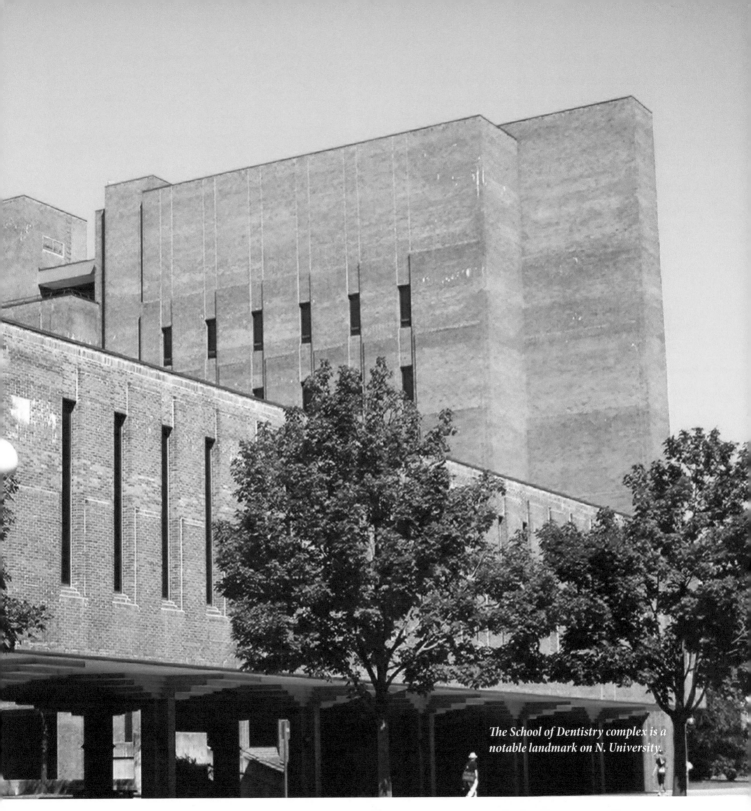

*The School of Dentistry complex is a notable landmark on N. University.*

Following the school's accreditation review in 1995, a Futures Committee was established to develop a plan whose cornerstone remained comprehensive care. The committee emphasized the need to get dental students into clinics earlier than their third or fourth year of dental school. Other key recommendations of the Futures Committee included expanding the comprehensive care approach to all four years of a dental student's clinical experience, having all dental hygiene students in the same clinics as dental students, and updating the curriculum so classroom instruction paralleled clinical experiences.[1]

This patient-centered approach to dental education was introduced as a pilot program and its success led to a major conference being held in Ann Arbor in November 1996. Representatives from dental schools, medical centers, insurance companies, organized dentistry, and the private sector met to discuss the challenges of implementing the new patient-centered curriculum. Favorable responses during the conference led to the decision to formally adopt this model and the launch of the Vertically Integrated Clinics (VICs) program the following June.[2]

## Vertically Integrated Clinics

The introduction of the VICs, as they were often called, was one of the biggest changes that occurred in the curriculum and patient care during the late 1990s. The VICs represented a sharp departure from previous models of dental education.

The VICs were a composite of several dynamics. "Vertical" represented a student's "moving up" through the dental program from the first through fourth years

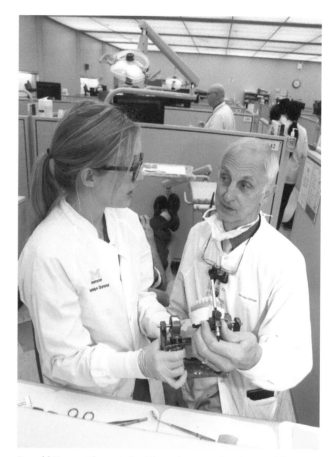

*Donald Heys guides a student through a procedure in one of the student clinics.*

and from the second through fourth years for dental hygiene students. Each year introduced activities of greater complexity with the expectation of increased levels of competence and the ability to take on more responsibility. The change was significant for dental hygiene students. Previously, they saw patients in a clinic separate from dental students and were only in clinic three mornings a week—Monday, Wednesday, and Friday. The VIC model allowed the dental hygiene students to participate in clinical activities five days a week and dental hygiene patients were seen in both morning and afternoon sessions.

The word "integrated" involved a team approach that offered a special package of patient-centered comprehensive care to each and every patient seen at the dental school. Dental and dental hygiene students benefited from this approach, as the learning environment was designed to more closely resemble the private-practice setting. Patients benefited because under the new model, care was based on their individual needs and delivered through treatment plans developed jointly by students, patients, and faculty.

Another advantage of the VIC model was that first-year dental students now had early access to the clinics. They actually could see what was going on in clinic from the day they entered dental school. Although first-year dental students did not treat patients, they were able to assist upperclassmen and learn the ins and outs of working in a dental environment that included clinical care, patient interactions, infection control, and record-keeping. First-year dental hygiene students, who started their dental school experience as sophomores, followed a similar path. While they spent time developing their skills in preclinic, they also spent time in clinic where they observed junior and senior students providing care and were able to perform simple procedures such as polishing or topical fluoride applications.

These early experiences were valuable because by the time the students began to treat their own patients, both dental and dental hygiene students knew a lot about clinical procedures, patient communications, and the importance of teamwork.

First-year dental students (D1s) were assigned to one of four comprehensive care clinics located on the second and third floors of the dental building. The clinics, named for the color of the dental chairs in each clinic—2 Blue, 2 Green, 3 Blue, and 3 Green—became the "clinical home" for each student throughout all four years of dental school. Clinical faculty members were assigned to the same clinic each year and thus could better assess the clinical progress of the students in their clinic. Care provided in the VICs included restorative/operative, prosthodontic, and periodontal procedures. Students participated in scheduled rotations to get experience in orthodontics, pediatric, and oral surgery.[3]

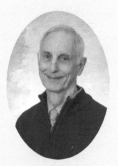

**Dr. Donald Heys** (DDS 1972, MS 1975), a professor in Cariology, Restorative Sciences and Endodontics and director of the 2 Blue Clinic, recalls the early years of the VICS:

*Dr. Donald Heys.*

The VICs model was very successful. Good things were happening and the faculty members involved were committed to its continuing success. One area we saw a big improvement in was an increase in the use of the clinical facilities compared to a few years earlier. We were thrilled to see clinic use at 90 to 95 percent.[4]

Even more important, was that this approach integrated didactic content being taught with the clinical procedures they were doing—each complementing the other. Students quickly realized how lectures and preclinical content made even more sense, because these things were taught in the context of the care they were providing in clinic.

Heys said:

> The VICs approach enriched the clinical experience for everyone. . . . Faculty members got to know their students and vice versa. That helped to develop rapport, understand a student's abilities, and identify where they needed a little more help. Our students were handling more complex cases and gaining invaluable clinical experiences while patients were receiving exceptional care. This also made it better for patients who, when returning for follow-up treatment, returned to the same clinic each visit.
>
> Patients with complex treatment plans required many appointments over an extended period of time. Because of this, students and patients often developed a special bond. Some patients even attended the commencement ceremonies to see their student graduate from dental school.[4]

Another administrator, **Dr. Lisa Tedesco**, associate dean for Academic Affairs, said VICs were important because "they helped move the school from a requirement-based approach to a learning-based one that emphasized patient-centered care. That approach was not just technical in nature. . . . It emphasized a focus on the complete patient clinically, including social factors that affected him or her." That included a better understanding of a patient's ethnicity, their personal and professional background, their education, overall health, and other experiences. "These were all a part of a total approach to care each patient would receive," Tedesco said.

## Technology's Growing Importance in Education and Patient Care

Dental and dental hygiene education was being enhanced with more information being offered in a new way—on the Internet. Recognizing the importance of strong information management skills for future health-care professionals, coursework was designed to actively engage students in the use of MEDLINE and other Internet searches, and to teleconference to work with faculty members and peers at other sites. A computer server was set up to house content that allowed students to access course syllabi, notes, and selected readings from school or home, as well as retrieve photos, charts, and radiographs for use in treatment planning exercises.[5] In 1996, the school announced the launch of its website, making access to School of Dentistry information for anyone interested just a few keystrokes away. Initially, the website content focused on material for students, prospective students, and those interested in continuing education offerings. Later, content was expanded to include general information about the school, department news, and alumni and development events.[6]

The growth of the Internet was extraordinary, with tens of thousands of people visiting the School of Dentistry website each month. In 1996, the National Library of Medicine funded a three-year project, led by Paul Lang, to assess the use of the Internet as a method of providing distance learning to dentists. Study participants were solicited from Michigan and throughout the United States. The school also offered its first completely online course. Ten fourth-year dental students participated in Information Management Issues for Dentistry 815 as a pilot program to determine whether a dental school course could be taught successfully online rather than as a standard series of lectures.[7] The results from this course and others that followed paved the way for the launch of the dental hygiene program's degree completion e-learning program in 2008. The program was the first online degree completion program offered by the University of Michigan (U-M) Ann Arbor campus.[8]

## Renovations and Facilities Enhancement

Significant renovations and improvements to existing physical facilities began, with major renovations to the Kellogg Building in 1997. Renovations were completed in 2000 at a cost of nearly $13 million, just in time for the celebration of school's the 125th anniversary.

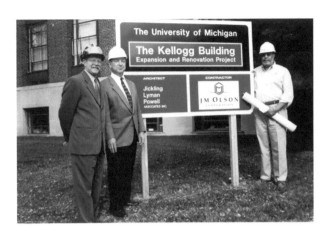

*Dean William Kotowicz (L) and Assistant Dean Arnold Morowa with Gary Owens (R) outside the Kellogg Building before the renovation project begins.*

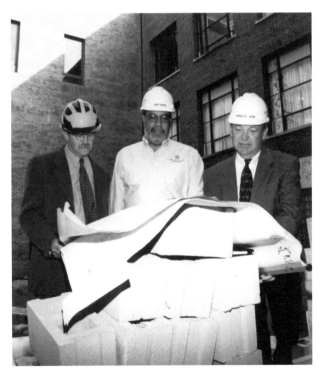

*Dean William Kotowicz (L) and Assistant Dean Arnold Morowa (R) confer with Gary Owens on the construction plans.*

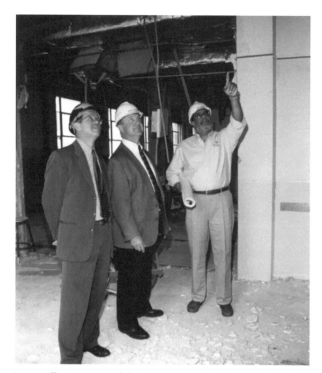

*Dean William Kotowicz (L) and Assistant Dean Arnold Morowa with Gary Owens (R) scan construction details during the Kellogg Building renovation project.*

A ceremony held in the new Sindecuse Atrium on September 8, 2000, celebrated the end of the Kellogg renovations, the naming of three new clinic areas for three distinguished alumni, the dedication of the new Sindecuse Atrium, and the 125th anniversary of the school's founding. Among those attending were U-M President Lee Bollinger and Provost Nancy Cantor.

## Three Facilities for Three Distinguished Alumni

The three clinical facilities that were part of the Kellogg renovation were the Robert W. Browne Orthodontic

Wing, the Kenneth A. Easlick Pediatric Dentistry Clinic, and the Samuel D. Harris Children's Dental Unit.

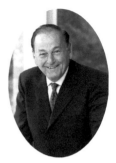

*Dr. Robert W. Browne*

Robert W. Browne (DDS 1952, MS Orthodontics 1959) gifted $1.5 million to the school for a new orthodontic clinic that, as he described, "probably has not been altered since I was a student."[9] A similar sentiment was voiced by Dr. James McNamara who was put in charge of renovations to the orthodontic clinic by Dr. Lysle Johnston, department chair. "The facilities we had been using were antiquated, at best," McNamara

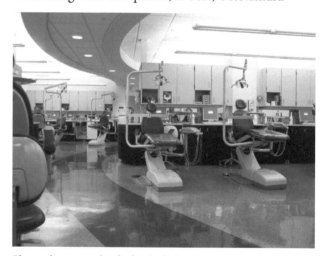

*The newly renovated orthodontic clinic.*

said. "The renovations were sorely needed." New orthodontic facilities included a patient waiting room, 34 dental chairs in an open clinic setting, complete radiographic facilities, new offices, and conference rooms.

Kenneth A. Easlick (DDS 1928), considered by many to be the father of pediatric dentistry,

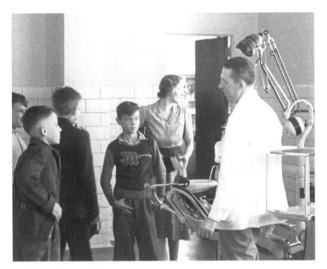

*Dr. Kenneth A. Easlick.*

developed the school's first teaching program in children's dentistry shortly after he earned his dental degree from Michigan in 1928. The pediatric dentistry clinic named for him included 22 chairs in a semi-open clinic setting for graduate student training, two quiet rooms for children with special needs, a graduate studies seminar room, and clinical outcomes research facilities.[10,11]

Samuel D. Harris (DDS 1924), known as the founder of the American Society of Dentistry for Children, dedicated his career to encouraging all segments of the dental profession—teachers, clinicians, general, pediatric, and public health dentists—to promote better dental health for all children. The children's dental

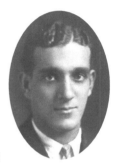

*Graduation photo of Samuel D. Harris, DDS 1924.*

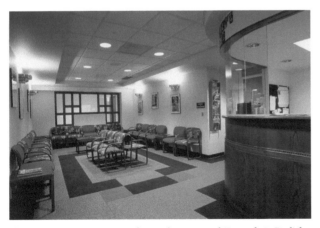

*The patient waiting room in the newly renovated Kenneth A. Easlick Pediatric Dentistry Clinic.*

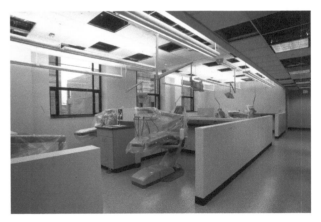

*New dental chairs still covered in plastic in the Samuel D. Harris Children's Dental Unit.*

**Artist Frances Danovich** said that in creating the mural, he "tried to convey simply an amusing and light fantasy, using the elements found in real lumber camps. . . . The mural is originally planned for children. But since adults too will see it, I have attempted to make it acceptable to a varied audience." Unfortunately, only portions of the mural could be salvaged. Today, there are three mural panels on exhibit in the Sindecuse Atrium.[14]

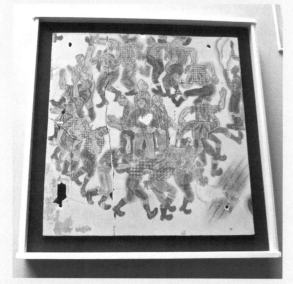

*One of the Danovich murals salvaged from the lobby of the children's clinic in the old dental building.*

A surprising discovery was made during the Kellogg Building renovations. The "Babe the Blue Ox" mural painted by Mr. Francis Danovich in the 1930s was found after it had been covered by wallpaper during the 1960s and forgotten. The mural was discovered as demolition was about to begin to make room for the Robert W. Browne Orthodontics Wing.

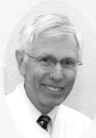

*Dr. Bud Straffon.*

Pediatric dentist **Dr. Lloyd "Bud" Straffon** (DDS 1963) lauded the finding of the "lost" mural:

Originally, the murals were in the lobby of the pediatric clinic and while children waited they talked about the mural and asked questions of their parents. That was how they entertained themselves and took their minds off of being seen by a dentist. . . . But times have changed. Today, kids may have video games they bring to entertain themselves while they wait. (Personal communication, April 9, 2015)

unit included 10 dental chairs for predoctoral student training, an updated instrument handling area, and a parent/patient consultation room. [12,13]

## From Courtyard to Atrium

Also included in the Kellogg project were updates to the Gordon H. Sindecuse Museum of Dentistry and

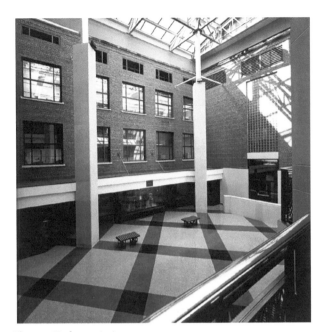

*The new Sindecuse Atrium.*

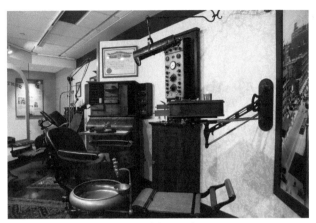

*One of the Sindecuse Museum exhibits in the new atrium.*

enclosing the adjacent open-air courtyard. Renovation of the Sindecuse Museum, which opened in 1992, featured more space for storage and exhibitions and climate controlled areas to help preserve dental equipment, photographs, and other memorabilia.[15] The new Sindecuse Atrium featured a glass roof covering the courtyard that now, protected from the elements, served as both exhibit space for the museum and event space for the school. The atrium can accommodate more than 200 people for luncheons and other special events, including those held during Homecoming Weekend.

Other renovations followed in 1998. Improvements were made to the student forum, officially named the Alpha Omega Fraternity Detroit Alumni Student Forum following a $50,000 gift to the school to support the project. Two new lecture rooms were built, one with 94 seats (G550) and the other with 36 seats (G580) were equipped with outlets that allowed students and faculty to connect their portable computers to the Internet. Elevated walkways offered access to the Kellogg Building from the first and second floors of the dental school building. Renovations also included clinics for endodontics, periodontics, and restorative dentistry, as well as restrooms that complied with the Americans with Disabilities Act, and enhancements to sterilization, dispensing, and records facilities. These costs, added to the $13 million spent on the Kellogg renovations, brought the construction costs for all projects to more than $20 million.[16]

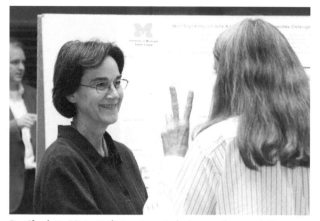

*Dr. Charlotte Mistretta listens to a student research presentation.*

## Research Renaissance

Changes were underway in the school's research activities. When he became dean, Kotowicz began to bolster the school-wide Oral Health Sciences (OHS)/PhD program. Citing the school's strong reputation for its master's and clinical programs, Kotowicz said the school did not have a well-defined, school-wide research and training program at the doctoral level, and he made that a priority. Dr. Charlotte Mistretta was asked to take on this challenge and her efforts helped to redefine the OHS/PhD program.

The OHS/PhD program was designed to strengthen basic, translational, clinical and health services research initiatives.

The fundamental goal of the program was to train exceptional students to become leaders in academic research, oral health maintenance, and disease prevention. Students were able to explore an array of biological, chemical, and physical aspects of oral health problems in six broad areas of study—craniofacial

development and anomalies, tissue engineering and regeneration, microbial diseases and immunity, mineralized tissue and musculoskeletal disorders, oral neuroscience, and oral and pharyngeal cancer.[17]

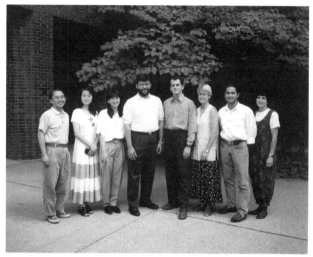

*Among the initial Oral Health Sciences/PhD cohort were (L–R) Hen-Li Chen (2002, dual degree MS and PhD student), Hongjiao Ouyang (2000), Somjin Ratanasathien (2000), Esam Tashkandi (1999), Jacques Nör (1999), Erika DeBoever (2001), Andre Haerian (2003), and Domenica Sweier (2004). Year of graduation is noted in parentheses.*

The first PhD degrees in OHS were conferred in 1999 to Jacques Nör and Esam Tashkandi.

## OHS/PhD—Three Options

The OHS/PhD program offered students three program options to help them achieve their goals. The first option available to those aspiring to a career in dental research was the original OHS/PhD program. A second option combined a clinical master's degree in a dental specialty while simultaneously pursuing the OHS/PhD. The third option was available to students whose goal it was to combine a DDS degree with a PhD in oral health research.

Mistretta said:

> Students who have completed this program have progressed to careers in research and academic dentistry. . . . Their success, in turn, is attracting other exceptional and highly-motivated students who want to "push themselves" to achieve even more, both professionally and personally.[18]

Kotowicz said the program has succeeded "because of Charlotte's ability to see the big picture and her ability to bring people together to achieve an objective."[19]

Wanting to broaden the school's research portfolio and secure more federal funding for research, Kotowicz named Dr. Christian Stohler as the school's research director in 1995.[20] Building on the success of Dr. Sigurd Ramfjord's research, faculty in the Department of Periodontics, Prevention and Geriatrics focused on reducing periodontal disease, regenerating and repairing oral hard and soft tissues, and applying discoveries in the basic sciences to help patients.[21]

Research in the Department of Oral Medicine, Pathology and Oncology focused on angiogenesis (the growth of blood vessels) and its relationship to cancer and other diseases. Faculty members in Cariology, Restorative Sciences and Endodontics began to put their efforts into clinical research studying dental materials and why restorations fail and participating in controlled clinical trials in private practice as well as health

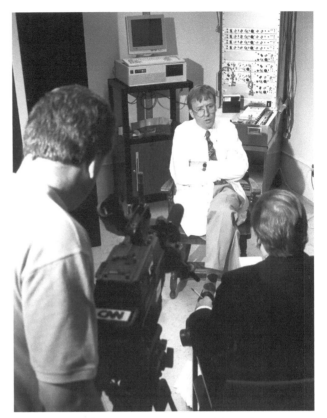

*Dr. Christian Stohler giving an interview to CNN on pain.*

services research. These studies moved the department into another research arena with huge implications for dental practice and evidence-based dentistry.[22]

"Translating" discoveries in research laboratories that could be used in dental clinics was the focus of a one-year grant to establish the Center for the Biorestoration of Oral Health (CBOH) in 1996. CBOH director Dr. Laurie McCauley said it was the new frontier for the school's research because it brought together dental, medical, biomedical, engineering, and other researchers to develop novel therapies that could improve the health and quality of life for patients with oral, dental, craniofacial, and other disorders. The center's focus was on regeneration biology and work in this area helped as a catalyst to bring many scientists together to collaborate and foster stronger projects in regenerative medicine and tissue engineering.[23]

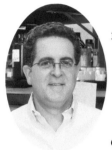

The focus on translational research was further promoted when Dr. Renny Franceschi was appointed director of research in 1998. He encouraged clinical research with the ultimate goal of moving basic findings into the clinic to promote health.

*Dr. Renny Franceschi*

## Scientific Frontiers in Clinical Dentistry

National Institute of Dental and Craniofacial Research (NIDCR) made history when, for the first time ever, it brought its Scientific Frontiers in Clinical Dentistry program to a college campus. On January 5 and 6, 2000, the U-M School of Dentistry hosted this prestigious program. Dr. Arnold Morawa, assistant dean for Alumni Relations and Continuing Dental Education, proposed the idea for the Michigan program in 1997 to Dr. Harold Slavkin, NIDCR director. "We planned to develop a program with a clinical focus," Morawa said. "Our objective was to give those who attended an opportunity to hear about laboratory research and show how science could be applied to clinical practice."[24]

More than 1,500 dental professionals from across the country came to Ann Arbor to listen to world-renowned clinicians and researchers discuss advances in dentistry and clinical research, and learn how this research benefits both practitioners and patients. U-M President Lee Bollinger delivered the opening remarks and outlined the university's new $200 million Life Sciences Initiative that called for building a state-of-the-art facility that would foster greater interdisciplinary collaboration in the life sciences and reposition the university as a leader in health and life sciences research and education.[25] By all measures, the program was a tremendous success and underscored a long-standing commitment Michigan had made to dentistry and dental science decades earlier.

Dr. Martha Somerman, who became associate dean for research in January 2001, said that at Michigan, research was essential. "There was always a commitment to education among the faculty to graduate the best practitioners possible. Research and knowledge gained from research guided the development of our education programs which

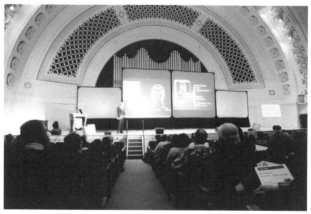

*More than 1,500 people from across the country participated in the Scientific Frontiers in Clinical Dentistry program hosted by the School of Dentistry.*

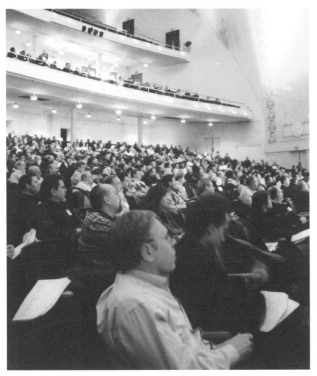

*Program participants listen to world-renowned clinicians and researchers discuss advances in dentistry and clinical research.*

focused on evidence-based scientific approaches to inform practice decisions," she said.

## Funding the Research Enterprise

Funding for the research enterprise grew. Per the data provided by the school's Office of Research and Research Training (Pat Schultz, personal communication, February 17, 2014) in 1997, the NIDCR awarded $4.9 million to the School of Dentistry. It increased to more than $8.5 million by the time Kotowicz's term as dean ended in 2003.

## With Success Comes Challenges

As the research enterprise grew, the need for additional space also grew. Research space in the dental school building was at capacity and beyond. The only option was to move some of its operations to off-campus sites. In 2002, several research activities were moved to the Eisenhower Commerce Center on the south side of Ann Arbor. Clinical billing and financial operations moved to the Arbor Lakes Commerce Center on Plymouth Road just outside Ann Arbor's northeast side.

## Outreach Expands

For many years, dental students provided oral health care to children during the Summer Migrant Dental Clinic program in the Traverse City area or at the Bay Cliff Health Camp northwest of Marquette. Pediatric residents also applied their knowledge and skills helping children in the Flint, Michigan, area. In July 1993, pediatric dental residents began providing oral health care as part of a relationship that involved the School of Dentistry's Mott Children's Health Center and Hurley Hospital.[26]

Dr. Jed Jacobson was named assistant dean for community and outreach programs in 1997. Not long after taking on this responsibility, Dean Kotowicz approached Jacobson and said, "I need you to take on a new responsibility." Jacobson recalls:

> Bill said he wanted to re-examine the school's model of education so that it would include having students provide dental care in

communities across Michigan for some part of the academic year. That was a tall order. Bob Bagramian and Marilyn Woolfolk did a wonderful job with outreach in the Traverse City area, but there was little, if any, funding for a larger effort that would include other communities across the state. (Personal Communication, July 23,2015)

Jacobson went straight to work to expand the program. The effort gained traction following meetings Jacobson had with Rick Bossard, government relations officer for the U-M Health System, and State Senator Joe Schwarz of Battle Creek. Public and private sector organizations collaborated to make the expanded outreach program a reality. They included the Michigan Department of Community Health, the Michigan Dental Association, the Delta Dental Fund (the philanthropic arm of Delta Dental), the Michigan Primary Care Association, the Michigan Campus Compact, the Josiah Macy Jr. Foundation, and the W.K. Kellogg Foundation's Civic Engagement Program.[27]

Although the Summer Migrant Dental Clinic program was nearly two decades old when she arrived at the School of Dentistry in July 1992 to become associate dean for Academic Affairs, Dr. Lisa Tedesco said that the program helped both the school and the university. "It was important because it elevated the school's visibility to Michigan citizens and was a model for other outreach efforts," she said.

In early 2000, under Jacobson's leadership and direction, the community outreach program emerged as a "year round" component of the dental education curriculum. Instead of taking place just in the summer, as it had for years, dental and dental hygiene students were now involved in community dentistry during the entire academic year (late summer to early spring of the following year) during their final year.

Dental students traveled to sites and worked alongside other oral health professionals in new locations—Grand Rapids, Battle Creek, Saginaw, Muskegon Heights, and Marquette. Dental students completed one-week rotations in three communities for a total of three weeks. Dental hygiene students participated in a single-week rotation. Residents in

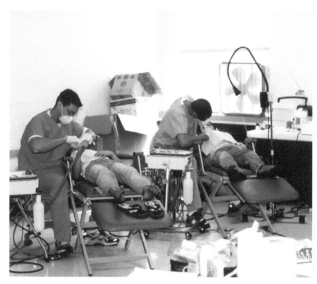

*Students gain valuable experience providing much needed care at the migrant dental clinics.*

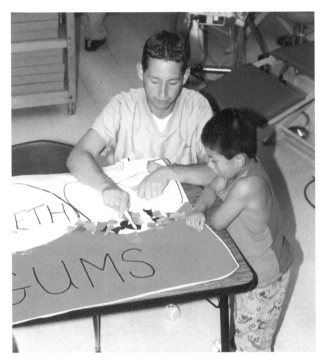

*Patients at the migrant dental clinic benefit from oral hygiene instruction with fun visual aids.*

specialty oral health-care programs and those in the Advanced Education in General Dentistry program were also involved.[28]

The enhanced program benefited students, providers, and patients in the five communities. Students often treated patients with conditions not typically seen in the dental school's on-campus clinics. The program allowed the students to live in communities throughout the state which improved the profile of U-M in those communities. Students also gained important insight into the communities they served. By working and living in the communities,

students also gained a better understanding of problems in those areas. The arrangement also allowed local oral health-care providers to have more patients treated at their facilities. Patients, many who had not received oral health care in years, now received the care they needed.

## Teaching with Technology

The school was being recognized for the innovative ways it was using new technology. In 2000, its Comprehensive Treating Planning website became a part of the Smithsonian's Permanent Research Collection on Information Technology housed at the National Museum of American History. The site, created by Drs. Dennis Fasbinder and Jeffery Shotwell, was the first of its kind at the school to use a "virtual patient," instead of 35-mm slides, to teach dental

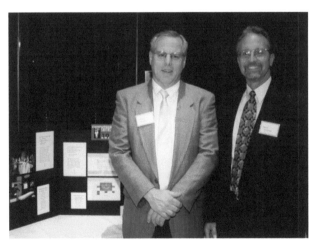

*Drs. Jeffery Shotwell (L) and Dennis Fasbinder at the Computerworld Awards presentation ceremony held October 5, 2000.*

students about the benefits of various oral health-care treatments.[29]

A year later, the school received the Computerworld Smithsonian Award that acknowledged developing novel uses of technology that benefit society. The school's winning entry, in the Education and Academic category, was an interactive movie designed to teach head and neck anatomy to dental and medical students. The head and neck anatomy movie was developed by Dr. John Lillie.[30]

By 2000, the school began digitizing images of microscopic sections of oral lesions. The project was an effort to make the images available for teaching and learning on the school's intranet, accessed by faculty, staff, and students by a special password. More than 10,000 slides were digitized and were available to help pathologists and clinicians in diagnosis, teaching, and collaboration. Digital technology continued to advance as orthodontics became the first department to move to an all-electronic, paperless clinical operation.

## A New Tradition

The White Coat Ceremony initiated a "new tradition" for the school. The first ceremony was held in the fall of 2002 and each of 105 first-year dental students was welcomed to the school and the dental profession. Each student was called by name to formally receive the white coat that they would wear during their dental education.

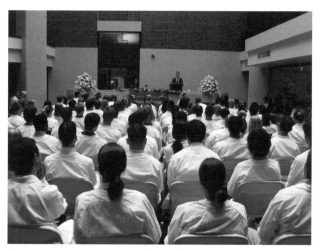

*First White Coat Ceremony held in Sindecuse Atrium on October 3, 2002. Dr. Philip Richards addresses the dental students.*

## Commitment to a Positive Workplace

The school's administrators were committed to insuring that the School of Dentistry was a welcoming and safe place for faculty, staff, students and patients to interact, learn, work, and be treated in a supportive manner. During the 1995 academic year, the school conducted its first multicultural audit to assess the climate for diversity and inclusion in the dental school. One of the recommendations in the audit's final report was to create a special committee, responsible for activities designed to promote change and monitor the progress made toward improving the multicultural climate in the school. The committee would be an advisory committee to the dean and provide annual progress reports.

To that end, Kotowicz formed the Multicultural Affairs Committee (MAC), made up of students, staff and faculty, charged with developing activities to advance excellence through diversity by exploring and celebrating differences and similarities among all groups. Led by Lisa Tedesco, associate dean for Academic Affairs, Cheryl Quiney, patient care coordinator, Patient Services, and Marita Inglehart, associate professor, Department of Periodontics and Oral Medicine, the MAC became the catalyst for change, cultivating a humanistic and collaborative environment that readily aligned with the school's strategic initiatives.

The **Multicultural Affairs Committee** has been active since it was formed in 1996. In 2017, the MAC celebrated 20 years of service to the school. Activities sponsored by the MAC include:

- Martin Luther King Jr. Day
- Women's History Month Tea
- The School of Dentistry Quilt Project
- Veterans Day Observance
- Ida Gray Awards
- Taste of Culture–The Taste Fest
- The Multicultural Mirror
- Schoolwide Cultural Audits
- Understanding Disabilities/Patients with Special needs—CE
- Getting to Know You—brown bag lunch sessions
- Diversity Sessions during D1 Orientation
- D1 Trip to the African American Museum in Detroit
- Unconscious Bias Workshops

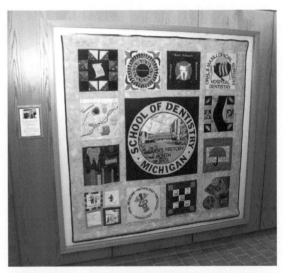

*Staff and faculty women artfully created this quilt in 2001 as part of the annual Women in History Month celebration. It symbolizes the diversity of the dental school community working together for the benefit of the patients and the public served.*

## Reflections

The Kotowicz years were years of change and transformation at the School of Dentistry. The "transition period" initiated a major reorganization effort reducing 18 academic departments to 6. Overall operations were decentralized; budget challenges were addressed; and cost centers were established for the programs. Academic and administrative collaborations were promoted and resource allocations were rethought. These strategies became a model for other schools and colleges at the U-M. Equally important was that the School of Dentistry no longer was isolated from the greater campus. It was now considered an integral part of the U-M. The success of these administrative and curricular changes were watched closely by dental schools around the country and became a standard to which others aspired.[31]

*Chapter 7*

# The Polverini Years (2003–2013)

In February 2003, University of Michigan (U-M) Regents approved the appointment of Dr. Peter Polverini as dean of the School of Dentistry. He assumed the position on June 1, 2003.[1]

Polverini, having just returned to U-M after serving three years as dean at the University of Minnesota, was keenly aware of the school's world-class reputation and long tradition of quality in all areas of its mission—education, research, and patient care. In conversations with the faculty, staff, students, and alumni, he stressed that his primary goal as dean was to embrace all three mission areas and use existing strengths as the foundation upon which to build a model of dental education, both forward thinking and sustainable.[2] This model would be informed by scientific discovery that would enrich the education students receive and enable them to deliver the very best patient care.

## Technology-Enhanced Education

Increasingly, technology was changing how students learned and how faculty taught. Prospective students began to evaluate not just a school's faculty and its programs, but also its technology and how that technology was being used. A survey of new dental students in the fall of 2002 revealed that slightly more than 40 percent said they owned a laptop computer.

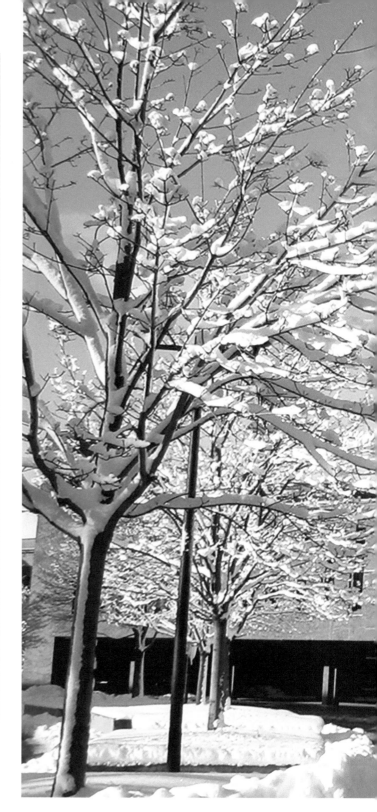

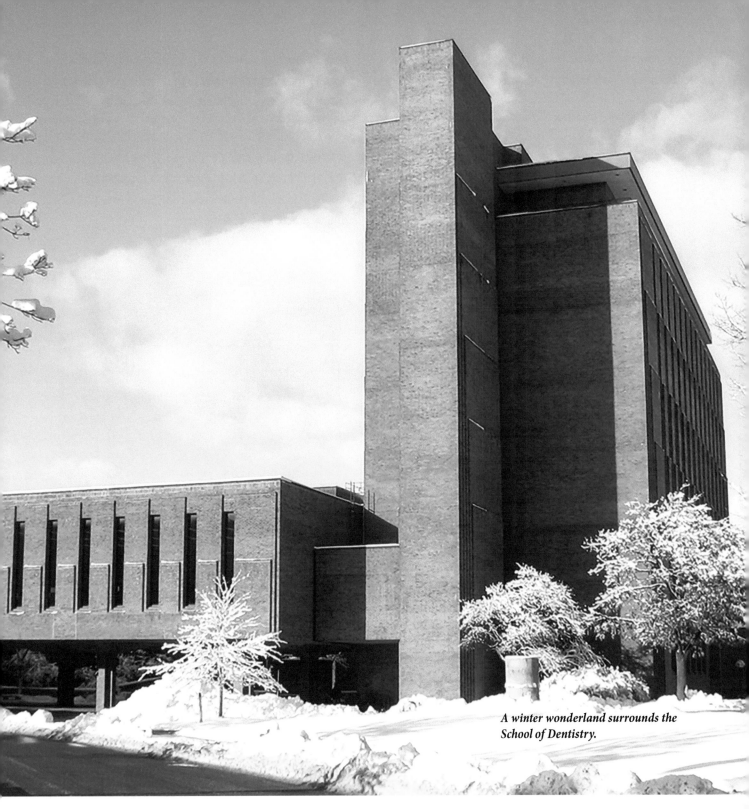

*A winter wonderland surrounds the School of Dentistry.*

Three years later, nearly two-thirds did.[3] Today, all dental students use laptops and various mobile devices.

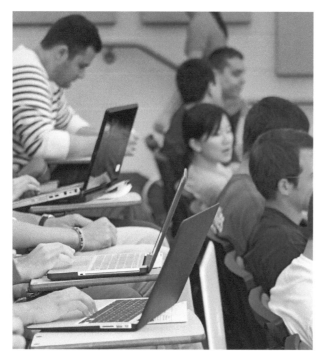

*Laptops have become an essential learning tool for students.*

A new era in preclinical dental education began in the summer of 2003 when the west wing of the old preclinical laboratory was gutted to make way for a new "high-tech clinic." The renovations, completed in January 2004, were the first updates to that facility since the new dental school was completed in 1969.[4]

The new simulation lab, funded in part by a generous gift from the Roy H. Roberts family, was equipped with 110 workstations where first- and second-year dental students spent many hours learning clinical procedures. Each workstation was set up with a flat-screen monitor to allow students to watch demonstrations of various dental procedures delivered to the screen via video, document camera, the Internet, or other media.

Each workstation was also equipped with a manikin head used to simulate a patient in a dental chair. The manikin setup helped teach correct ergonomic positioning of both patient and clinician as well as the clinical procedures students learn.[4]

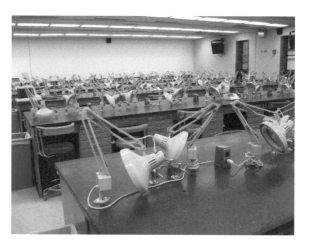

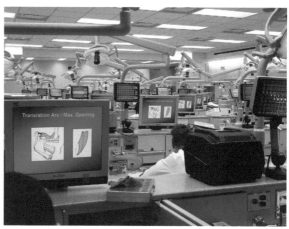

*The old preclinical laboratory (top) juxtaposed with the new.*

The preclinical lab is always part of the tour during the school's Homecoming Weekend celebration. Many alums have been heard to describe the facility as a technical marvel. Some have even said that many of the materials and techniques dental students were taught would have been science fiction to a new dental student three or four decades ago.

## Podcast—2005 Word of the Year

Always ahead of the curve, in 2004, second-year dental student Jared Van Ittersum (DDS 2008) approached the director of Dental Informatics, Dr. Lynn Johnson, and proposed that classroom lectures be recorded so dental students could download lectures to their computers or transfer the information to a laptop or some other portable device. This approach would allow them to review content and listen to the lectures at their convenience anywhere and at any time. This technology was called *podcasting* and the word "podcast" was tagged by the *New Oxford American Dictionary* as the 2005 Word of the Year.[5]

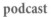 **podcast**

noun: A digital audio file made available on the Internet for downloading to a computer or mobile device, typically available as a series, new instalments of which can be received by subscribers automatically.

Working together, the Dental Informatics team and Van Ittersum, launched the podcasting initiative. The School of Dentistry was the first unit on the U-M campus and the first dental school in the country to

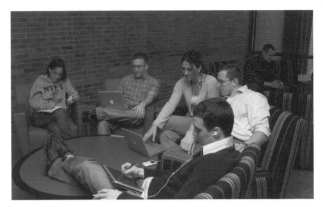

*Among the students participating in the podcasting program were members of the Class of 2008: (L–R) Elise Boncher, Patt Palazzolo, Sarah Miller, Adam Osga, and Justin Pearson.*

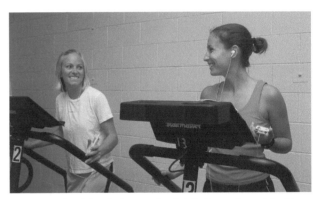

*Katie Beougher (L) and Elise Boncher (R), both members of the Class of 2008, listen to podcast lectures while working out at the Central Campus Recreation Building.*

podcast lectures, both record them and make them available to be downloaded. The student-led initiative was embraced by school administrators and also caught the attention of executives from Apple Computer. In September 2005, Apple Computer executives came to the School of Dentistry to personally congratulate the school for its novel use of technology.[6] Faculty members were given the choice to "opt out" of the lecture capture system, but few did. By the spring of 2007, the number of classroom lectures that dental students could listen to as podcasts surpassed 1,000. Since making this learning option available, dental students have accessed these lectures more than 30,000 times to listen to those lectures.[7]

## Outreach Expands—Again

Podcast technology was a tremendous help to dental students on outreach rotations across the state of Michigan. Since the number of outreach sites was growing and the length of time spent at a site was increasing, being able to access lecture content while away from the dental school was hugely important to the students. Appointed as director of outreach and community affairs in 2006, Dr. Bill Piskorowski worked diligently to add more clinics to the outreach milieu. A program that started with two sites, Adrian and Stockbridge, in 1970 eventually grew to 30 sites that included Federally Qualified Health Centers, tribal health authorities, private practices, hospitals, and community clinics. And from a week-long summer experience, time committed to rotations had increased to 3, then 4, and ultimately 12 weeks per student throughout the third and fourth years.

Although the time allotted to community-based clinical outreach experiences has varied over the years, patients across Michigan have consistently benefited from the care they have received. From May 2004 through March 2017, more than 172,000 patients had been seen statewide and nearly 319,250 procedures

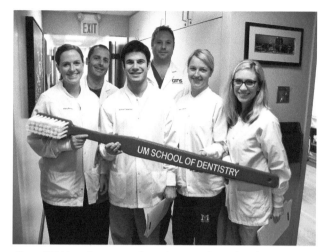

*Class of 2012 student outreach participants: (L–R, front): Hillary Mendillo, Michael Liberman, Jenna Comstock, and Lindsey Steele with Grand Traverse Health Clinic volunteer dentists (back left) Daniel Madion and Craig Fountain.*

were performed by U-M dental students with the value of those procedures estimated at more than $38 million.[8]

## Developing Future Leaders

The school has a long tradition of producing leaders whether they are students, faculty, or alums. Formal efforts to develop leadership skills among U-M dental and dental hygiene students began in August 2006 with the launch of a new program, the Scholars Program in Dental Leadership. Led by Dr. Russell Taichman, the program brought together a select number of exceptional students from diverse backgrounds to help cultivate a leadership mind-set and nurture skills they would later be able to use to effect change in their profession and in their communities.

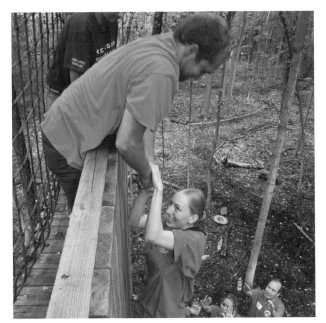

*Scholars Program in Dental Leadership (dental scholars) "kicks off" at the University of Michigan "Ropes Course" in August 2006. D1 Ben Anderson helps D3 Erica Scheller reach the top of a 13-foot wall. Below, other students and faculty extend their arms to cushion her if she slips. Goal was to get students to collaborate and devise a plan to get to the top. The wall was a metaphor for the obstacles or challenges they all will face.*

## Leaders and Best

The School of Dentistry has a long tradition of developing leaders and best in all aspects of dentistry. U-M dental alumni have served as leaders in education, clinical care, research, and professional organizations. And none more prominent than service to the profession through organized dentistry.

Records from the Michigan Dental Association (MDA) show more than 40 U-M graduates serving as MDA president starting in the early 1900s and continuing on through to Michele Tulak-Gorecki (DDS 1990) 2017–2018 term in office. Appendix C has a list of all MDA presidents who are U-M graduates.

Of special note is that three alums rose through the ranks of local and state leadership to reach the pinnacle of professional governance, president of the American Dental Association (ADA). Paul Jeserich (DDS 1924) served as the 1939–1940 MDA president and the 1959–1960 ADA president. Floyd Ostrander (DDS 1934, MS Endodontics 1941) served as the 1956–1957 MDA president and then as the 1967–1968 ADA president. Raymond Gist (DDS 1966) was elected the 2003–2004 MDA president and then ADA president, fulfilling the duties of that esteemed office in the 2010–2011 term.

Jeserich joined the School of Dentistry faculty in 1933. Committed to the highest standards of technical proficiency in clinical dentistry he directed the operative dentistry clinic for 11 years, from 1935 to 1946. In 1937 he assumed responsibility for directing the graduate and postgraduate programs sponsored by the W. K. Kellogg Foundation Institute, a position he held until his retirement. He was appointed dean in 1950 and served in that capacity until stepping down in 1962. He is recognized as an educator dedicated to the professional excellence of all School of Dentistry graduates and for his social concern for the general availability of dental care, working on behalf of the Ann Arbor Veterans Hospital and the Joint Council of the Health Professions to Improve the Health Care of the Aged.

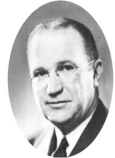

*Dr. Paul Jeserich*

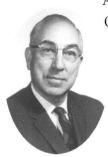

*Dr. Floyd Ostrander*

A professor of dentistry for 36 years, Ostrander was a widely known and highly regarded educator. He was an early promoter of the use of fluoride in toothpaste, helped establish endodontics as a specialty, and coauthored the internationally recognized textbook *Clinical Endodontics (1956, 1961, 1966)*. His training as a teacher, proficiency as a clinician, expertise in endodontics, and work with dental therapeutics gained him acclaim as one of the most influential and effective dental educators of his time. He also maintained a private practice in Ann Arbor until he retired in 1981.[9]

Gist was the youngest of eight children—the last born but the first in his family to attend college. Graduation from dental school was celebrated passionately throughout his community and "the pride that I felt from my family and community made me more determined than ever to be successful," Gist recalled. He went on to note,

> Dental school was no cake walk, but after completing the four challenging, intense, fun, and trying years in dental school, I recognized the investment the School of Dentistry had made in me; an investment that set me on a life changing career path.

> The skills and values I learned in dental school helped me become an excellent

clinician and laid the foundation for the leadership opportunities that followed, culminating in my election to the presidency of the ADA, 43 years after Dr. Ostrander.

Gist was the first African American president of the ADA. As ADA president, Gist was able to travel nationally and internationally. Gist said:

> I used my education and experience to promote, advocate, and educate the general public, and policymakers, about the benefits of good oral health and the challenges of providing it for all citizens. I learned that being proactive in gaining and maintaining a position at the forefront of my profession paid significant dividends, and it continues to do so.

Gist, who resides in Grand Blanc, Michigan, continues to serve the School of Dentistry and the university. He is active in the school's Profile for Success, a program for college students from disadvantaged and underrepresented backgrounds to be successful applicants for dental school. He makes frequent trips to Ann Arbor to work with the DDS students he mentors and to attend meetings of the Board of Directors of the U-M Alumni Association. (Personal Communication, August 2, 2017)

*Dr. Raymond Gist*

## Strategic Assessment and Strategic Imperatives

In 2005, U-M Provost Teresa Sullivan charged all U-M schools and units with the task of conducting a "clear-eyed" evaluation of their intellectual directions and priorities, strengths and weaknesses, comparative advantages over other schools, and value to the university. This charge triggered a significant strategic assessment process that culminated in a comprehensive strategic implementation plan for the School of Dentistry.

The strategic assessment process was led by a committee of 21 faculty, staff, and students. One of the guiding principles was to conduct an inclusive and dynamic systematic review of all School of Dentistry programs, units, and operational issues. The self-assessment took two years to complete and involved nearly every member of the School of Dentistry community. Input was received from internal and external review committees and the outcomes were published in a 27-page report in February 2007 entitled "Strategic Assessment of the School of Dentistry."

Synthesis of the Strategic Assessment Report formed the basis for the development of a set of strategic imperatives outlining a *vision* for the future of the dental school. The vision for the future included developing a new model for clinical education, investing in new technology to support the education and clinic programs, targeting growth of the research enterprise, and making a commitment to revitalize the research and patient care facilities.

With the emerging science of genomics and proteomics and the implications this knowledge would have on individualized treatments, it was imperative that dental graduates be prepared for a rapidly changing health-care environment. The key to success would be to develop a model for dental education that established linkages between research, education, and patient care.

## Culture and Climate

The School of Dentistry's leadership has always been very forward thinking in its effort to create a climate in which students, staff, faculty, and patients can interact, learn, work, and be treated in a supportive manner.

This was clearly demonstrated when, in 1973, Dean William Mann established the Office of Minority Affairs, dedicated to the recruitment of

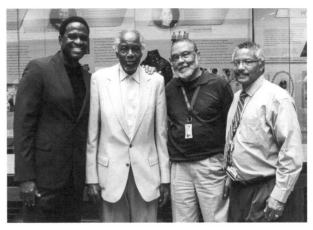

*Leaders, past and present, of the school's diversity and inclusion initiative: Drs. Todd Ester (1999–2006 and 2014–present), Lee Jones (1973–1996), Emerson Robinson (1996–1999), and Kenneth May (2007–2013).*

## Shaping the future—Vision for the School of Dentistry

- *Educational Program:* Transform the dental hygiene, predoctoral, and graduate educational programs (i.e., both clinical and biomedical sciences components) such that they serve as role models for dental education in innovation and financial sustainability.

- *Research:* Enhance the existing internationally recognized research enterprise such that the school has unquestioned preeminence in specific research focus areas.

- *Space and Facilities:* Implement short- and long-range plans to renovate, maintain, and increase academic, patient care, and research spaces, where feasible.

- *Faculty Funding:* Establish a new, sustainable funding model for faculty that is less dependent on general funds and provides significant opportunities for financial incentives.

- *External Influence:* Expand marketing strategies to ensure that U-M School of Dentistry is recognized across the state of Michigan, nationally and internationally as an outstanding resource for its education, research, patient care, and community service.

- *Culture and Climate:* Enhance all dimensions of diversity, multiculturalism, and professionalism so that the school environment is recognized, both internally and externally, as an exemplary place to study, work, and serve.

diverse students, staff, and faculty. This office evolved into the Office of Multicultural Affairs in 1999, the Office of Multicultural Affairs and Recruitment Initiatives in 2008, and the Office of Diversity and Inclusion since 2014.

The first school-wide multicultural audit was conducted in 1995. A follow-up audit was completed in 2007 to assess change over time. The outcomes of these audits guided the school leadership in their support of diversity initiatives at all levels (recruitment, retention, education, communication, and work–life balance). The ultimate goals were to ensure diversity, develop cultural competence, and improve the multicultural climate throughout the school.

## The Staff Forum

Staff employees are essential to School of Dentistry operations. They are often the unsung heroes who provide invaluable support to the faculty, the leadership, and students as they work to advance the vision and strategic mission of the school.

Over the years, both faculty and student groups had established a way to communicate issues to the dean and other school leaders. Staff employees, however, had no such mechanism. In an effort to ensure an inclusive work environment with open communication to all members of the School of Dentistry community, Dennis Lopatin (senior associate dean) and Tina Pryor (director of human resources) created the Staff Forum. The Staff Forum was formed to bring together a group of staff employees representing a cross section of all departments and units. The mission of the Staff Forum was to help facilitate an environment that promotes professional development and communications to enhance staff morale.

As they listened to the members of the Staff Forum talk about the issues staff were facing, Lopatin and Pryor came up with the idea of hosting a school-wide staff retreat. The first staff retreat was held in the spring of 2007. The half-day session featured a keynote speaker, followed by two or three breakout sessions. It was offered once in the morning and once in the afternoon to accommodate as many of the 330 staff people as possible. Everyone was invited to lunch.

The retreat was a huge success and feedback featured comments like "it is nice to see that leadership cares about us" and "this event demonstrates that the administration sincerely values our contributions to the School of Dentistry."

Subsequently, three additional "all staff" retreats were held (2009, 2012, and 2016) and the staff's participation has been phenomenal. All of the retreats have included sessions targeted at both professional and personal development. Topics offered encourage work life balance and well-being, time management, exercise and relaxation, quality communication, teamwork, meditation/relaxation, building trust and respect, and managing stress.

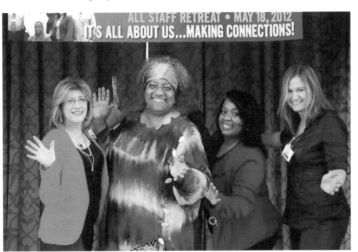

*Staff Forum—All Staff Retreat planners Gloria Sdao, Cheryl Quiney, Tina Pryor and Diane Thomas celebrating the success of the retreat.*

It is important to note that the School of Dentistry was the first school or college to host this type of "all school" staff activity on the U-M campus.

## Building a New Curriculum

To ensure that the school was going to remain among "the leaders and the best," the school leadership team determined that tackling the DDS curriculum was an important priority. All agreed it was time to update the curriculum with more contemporary educational strategies, strategies that would expand the students' experiences and enrich learning while simultaneously enhancing clinical knowledge to enable students to deliver the highest quality, patient-centered oral health care to an increasingly diverse and multicultural population.

Of significance was the belief that rapid advancement of scientific discovery and the desire to translate these findings to improved health care required a knowledge base that was well beyond what current dental graduates were expected to know. Therefore, the new curriculum would integrate science and clinical practice throughout all four years of dental school and new pedagogical methods to foster integration would be developed.

The need for a deeper understanding of the scientific underpinnings of dentistry was just one piece of the puzzle. There was also the need to cultivate

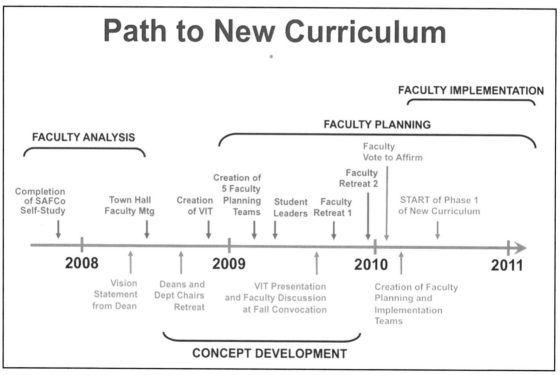

*Graphic from page 9, "Report to the School of Dentistry Community" prepared by the Vision Implementation Team.*

critical thinking and decision-making skills in all aspects of dental care. There was also a strong desire to offer a curriculum with flexible learning tracks providing expanded professional opportunities.

A Vision Implementation Team (VIT) was formed in 2008 and was charged to put in place a structure and path to enable faculty members to develop a new curriculum model that included (a) an enhanced teaching and learning environment that results in student independent decision-making and critical thinking, (b) development of new, flexible learning pathways that provide for expanded professional opportunities, and (c) better use of limited financial resources in the future. The VIT's major role was to facilitate planning and implementation of the vision by the faculty.

Members of the VIT were Paul Krebsbach (chair, Biologic and Materials Sciences, team chair), Stephen Bayne (chair, Cariology, Restorative Sciences and Endodontics), Dennis Lopatin (senior associate dean), Charlotte Mistretta (research dean), Jacques Nör (Cariology, Restorative Sciences and Endodontics), and Phil Richards (Periodontics and Oral Medicine). The team met faithfully every week for almost two years with a focus on developing a new curriculum. Their diligence and dedication delivered a new, innovative curriculum designed to produce a graduate grounded in scientific evidence, able to apply critical thinking and problem-solving skills in all aspects of oral health-care delivery—diagnosis, risk assessment, treatment planning, and clinical care.

## The New Curriculum Launches

In July 2010, the new, innovative dental curriculum was launched and introduced changes in preclinical instruction, earlier clinical experiences, opportunities for students to explore more career path options, greater collaboration with faculty, and more exposure to scientific knowledge needed in providing patient care. At the time, traditional dental curricula were linear in their staged presentation of basic science, clinical science, clinical procedures, clinical practice, and electives. The new curriculum started all of these phases simultaneously and carried them throughout the entire four-year experience.

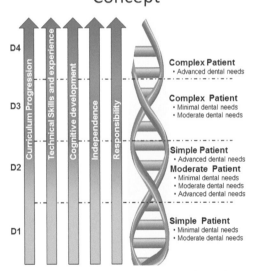

*Patient care progresses in levels of difficulty as students advance through the curriculum. Graphic from page 22,"Report to the School of Dentistry Community" prepared by the Vision Implementation Team.*

This integrated approach reinforced basic sciences with clinical content and introduced patient care experiences in the first year. At the same time, dental students were able to select a special area of interest or career path to explore in depth. In addition, a new concept called "flexible time" was built into each week. Flexible time was unscheduled time provided to students to allow them to absorb information conveyed in classrooms and clinics as well as facilitate opportunities to foster greater interaction among their colleagues and faculty.[10]

## The Pathways Program

The Pathways program offered every dental student a framework from which to explore a topic of personal interest in one of three distinct areas—health-care delivery, leadership, and research. Students work with faculty throughout their four years in dental school and engage in different types of scholarship

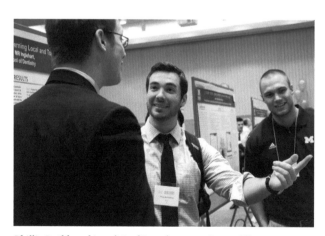

*Phillip Ruthkowski explains his pathways project to fellow students.*

In April 2012, as part of the leadership pathway, the **Wolverine Patriot Project** (WPP) was established. This project provided free, comprehensive dental care to disabled and homeless veterans in the Gaylord, Michigan, area. Led by dental student Jesse Edwards, students in the WPP saw an urgent oral health-care need that was not being met and did something about it. Two School of Dentistry alumni who practice in Gaylord, Dr. Edward Duski and his wife Dr. Janis Chmura Duski, allowed dental students to use their private practice office to treat the veterans under their supervision, many of whom reside in Gaylord at Patriot Place, a temporary residence for homeless veterans. During the first clinic, more than 40 veterans received oral health care, many for the first time in decades. Dental students returned to Gaylord monthly to provide oral health care during the weekend.

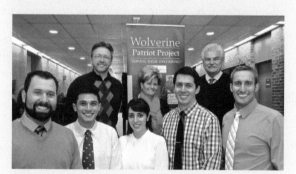

*Wolverine Patriot Project leaders: (L–R, front row) dental students Jesse Edwards, Kevin Goles, Mariam Dinkha, Ameen Shahnam, and Tony Guinn; (back row) Drs. Edward Duski, Janis Chmura Duski, and Bill Piskorowski (assistant dean of Community-Based Dental Education).*

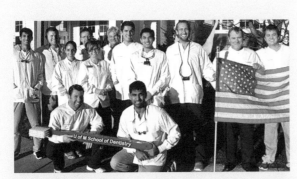

*A proud group of participant clinicians gather after providing dental care to veterans in Gaylord, Mich. The clinic was part of the 2012 Wolverine Patriots Project, a student-led, veterans-focused oral health initiative.*

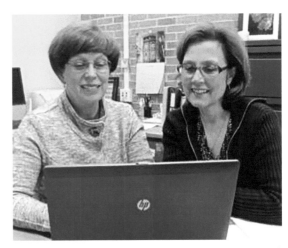

*Anne Gwozdek and Janet Kinney review the progress of the dental hygiene online learning students.*

through supplemental learning opportunities and capstone projects, depending on which pathway they choose. The program culminates with a special Pathways Day program where D4 students present summaries of the projects they have completed.

The first Pathways Day program was held in 2014 with the students presenting oral and poster summaries of their project and featured Ari Weinzweig (Zingerman's cofounder) as the keynote speaker.

## Dental Hygiene E-Learning

The use of technology to enhance education took a big step forward in January 2008 when the school launched its first online degree completion program leading to a Bachelor of Science in dental hygiene.

Eight students enrolled in the first cohort. The e-learning program attracted interest across U-M and from other colleges and universities worldwide. Dental hygiene students from around the country who earned an associate's degree or certificate were now able to take online courses at home or elsewhere, at their convenience, to earn a Bachelor of Science degree.[11,12]

The success of this program led to the development of a second online learning program, a Master of Science degree in dental hygiene, a two-year, six-semester course of study totaling 36 credit hours offered by the Rackham Graduate School in conjunction with the School of Dentistry. Professor Wendy Kerschbaum, director of the dental hygiene curriculum, said, "The online bachelor's degree program gave us a solid foundation that helped us to develop the master's program."[13]

## Hall of Honor

During Homecoming Weekend 2003, the school unveiled its Hall of Honor. A collaborative effort involving the school's Office of Alumni Relations and the Alumni Society Board of Governors, it recognizes and honors the achievements of dental profession legends, all deceased, who were associated with the U-M School of Dentistry during their lifetimes. The inaugural class included 18 men and women. By the fall of 2015, 47 men and women had been inducted into the Hall of Honor.

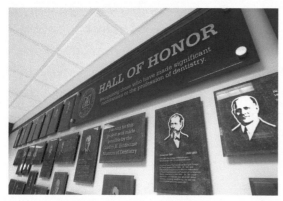

*A view of the University of Michigan School of Dentistry's Hall of Honor. (Photo by U-M Photo Services.)*

## Sindecuse Museum

In 2004, the museum's new curator, Shannon O'Dell, led efforts to create new exhibits including *Inside the Dental Practice, 1860–1940*, which highlighted the school's role in advancing dentistry, and *Women Dentists: Changing the Face of Dentistry*, which featured the achievements of more than 60 women who had a major impact on the profession.

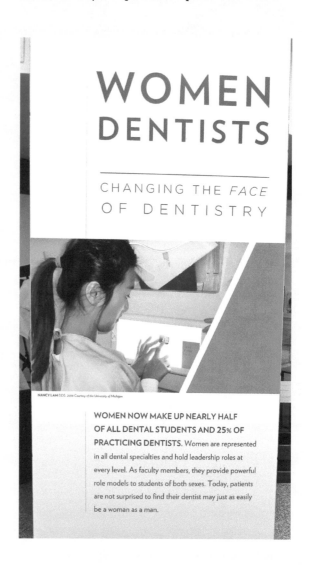

WOMEN DENTISTS

CHANGING THE *FACE* OF DENTISTRY

NANCY LAM DDS, 2008 *Courtesy of the University of Michigan*

**WOMEN NOW MAKE UP NEARLY HALF OF ALL DENTAL STUDENTS AND 25% OF PRACTICING DENTISTS**. Women are represented in all dental specialties and hold leadership roles at every level. As faculty members, they provide powerful role models to students of both sexes. Today, patients are not surprised to find their dentist may just as easily be a woman as a man.

## Electronic Patient Records

With the success of the transition from paper to an all-electronic environment in the orthodontic clinic, the school continued to embrace the electronic age when 160 computers were installed in the comprehensive care clinics (the VICs) on the second and third floors so that special software delivered patient information chairside with the touch of a few keystrokes. This advancement marked the fusion of innovation in technology, dental education, and patient care. The paper-to-digital transition was celebrated with a "floss-cutting ceremony" attended by U-M Provost Teresa Sullivan in June 2008.[14]

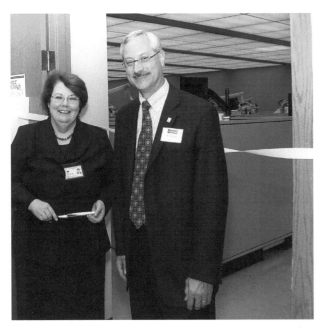

*Provost Teresa Sullivan and Associate Dean for Patient Services Stephen Stefanac prepare for the floss-cutting ceremony commemorating the launch of the electronic patient records in the clinics.*

## Provost: "I'm a Patient Here Too"

After complimenting the School of Dentistry for its innovative uses of technology, U-M Provost Teresa Sullivan also surprised some when she said, "I'm a patient here, too."

Sullivan, who had been U-M Provost for two years, said she receives oral health care in the Dental Faculty Associates Clinic. "It's the only dental service I use," she said after the floss-cutting ceremony. "The School's location is perfect for me given my responsibilities. It's convenient and it's state of the art."[14]

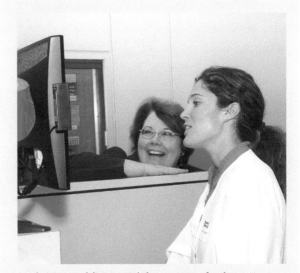

*Lindsey Wurtzel (DDS 2009) demonstrates the electronic patient record to Provost Teresa Sullivan.*

## The Dental Library Transforms

Since its founding, the dental library had always had its home in the School of Dentistry building. But things were rapidly changing. Libraries and librarians were among the first to embrace the information age using computer searches to assist faculty and students in their quest to locate materials available online. With the prevalence of digital content and electronic access to the content, many of the dental library's holdings were also digitized. In 2008, it was decided to merge the dental library with the Taubman Medical Library (renamed the Taubman Health Sciences Library in April 2010) and house both contemporary and historical holdings there. Much of dentistry's content is available online and those items physically stored at the health sciences library are conveniently accessible to researchers and others near and far.

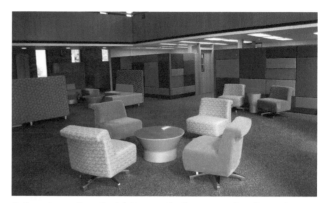

*Soft seating and a colorful decor make for a great place for students to gather.*

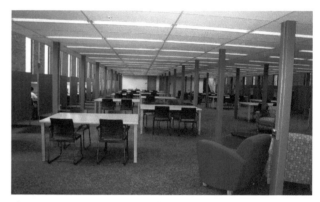

*The Commons—a quiet, comfortable place to study.*

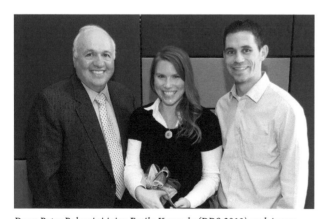

*Dean Peter Polverini joins Emily Kennedy (DDS 2013) and Aaron Ruhlig (DDS 2014) for the ribbon-cutting ceremony marking the opening of "The Commons" study area.*

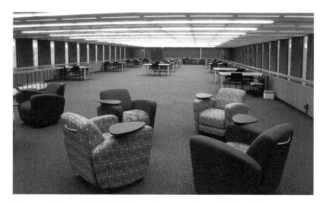

*More seating and study table on the upper level of The Commons.*

Not only was the library a repository for books, journals, course materials, and other reference items, it was also a great place for students to go to study. Students expressed concern that they had now lost their quiet study area. Responding to the students' concern, the library space was reconfigured, refurnished, and renamed "The Commons" in 2012. It is a very popular study space for students and also serves as home for the school's Human Resources Service Center.

## Old Technology, New Format

The school found new ways to use educational videos made in its television studios during the 1970s. More than 1,000 videos were changed to a digital format and became a part of the Open Michigan initiative designed to share the university's and the school's knowledge, resources, and research worldwide. The videos are a part of the university's YouTube Channel (www.youtube.com/user/umichdent).[15] According to Dan Bruell, director of the school's Digital Learning Services unit, by the fall of 2015, the videos had been viewed more than 20 million times worldwide. The most viewing occurred in the United States (28%), followed by India (10%), the United Kingdom (3.5%), Canada (3.5%), and Saudi Arabia (2.9%). The most watched video has been "Removal of Carious Lesions," viewed nearly 1.4 million times.

## Global Initiatives

The school formally committed to international outreach when the Global Oral Health Initiative program was created in 2011, and Dr. Yvonne Kapila was named program director. This new program was established to parallel U-M President Mary Sue Coleman's Third Century Initiative that sought to develop new avenues of learning and immerse students in experiences beyond campus classrooms. The school's initial efforts were sharply focused and built on established relationships in Ghana, Kenya, and Brazil. Over the years, many dental students have said participating in an international outreach experience has been the highlight of their four years of dental studies at Michigan.

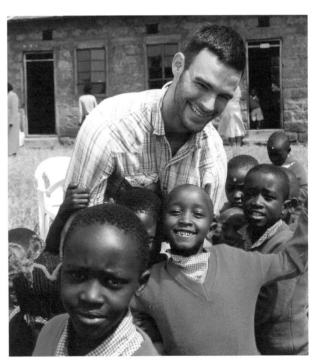

*Daniel Valicevic (DDS 2014), a 2012 participant in the Kenya Summer Research Program, is surrounded by lots of happy faces at a primary school in Meru, Kenya.*

## Interprofessional Education

Interprofessional education gained momentum during this time. Beginning in early 2012, school administrators and faculty led discussions with those from other units on campus to explore and implement a new approach to education. This approach encouraged all of the health sciences schools to rethink the traditional "siloed" method of education and patient care. Instead, the schools were encouraged to develop programs that involved students from multiple health-care professions—medicine, dentistry, public health, nursing, pharmacy, and social work— learning with, about, and from each other. One of the early pilots of this approach was implemented that summer. Students in the School of Nursing's Second Career Bachelor of Science program shadowed dental

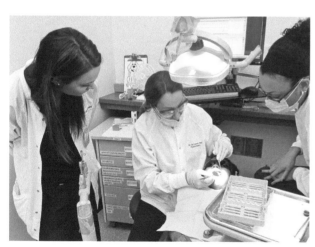

*As part of the interprofessional education initiative, Dr. Gail Czarnecki, clinical assistant professor, Department of Orthodontics and Pediatric Dentistry, developed a dental-focused program to allow nursing students to shadow dental students, residents, and faculty dentists in the pediatric dental clinic.*

students, residents, and faculty dentists in the dental school's pediatric dentistry clinic. The dental course was added to the School of Nursing's curriculum to familiarize nurses about oral health-care issues they may encounter in patients they see in various patient care situations.[16]

## Research Enterprise Flourishes

This era was marked by significant research grants from the National Institute of Dental and Craniofacial Research (NIDCR). Pat Schultz, administrative manager of the Office of Research and Training, said:

> Our research awards have been impressive. . . . During the 10 years from 2004 to 2013, NIDCR annually awarded the school between $8.6 million and $11.4 million for research. In three of those years (2006, 2009, 2011), the school ranked first among all dental schools in the country receiving awards. In four years (2004, 2005, 2008, 2013) the school ranked second. In 2007 and 2012, it ranked third. (Personal Communication February, 17, 2014)

Polverini said the awards were vital because research leads to discoveries that have the potential to benefit practitioners and their patients while also helping to advance the dental profession.[17] Collaborative research with other units on campus gained momentum when the school moved some of its research facilities to the North Campus Research Center in August 2012.

## Reflections

The Polverini era was a time of curricular change and transformation, and an expansion of technology used for teaching and data management. It was also at the time that saw significant growth of the research enterprise. A dynamic and determined faculty and staff committed to a new model for dental education that became a model for dental schools around the world endeavor to emulate.

Polverini received one of U-M's top honors in May 2015 when he was named the Jonathan Taft Distinguished University Professor of Dentistry. Distinguished University Professorships recognize individuals for major contributions to the university, the nation, and the world and for exceptional scholarly and/or creative achievements, national and international reputation, superior teaching and mentoring, and an impressive record of service.[18]

*Chapter 8*

# The McCauley Years (2013–)

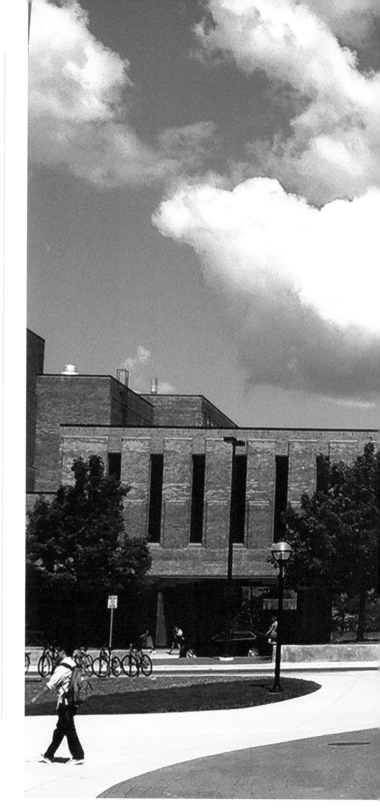

Following a national search, Dr. Laurie McCauley became the first woman and the 14th person to become dean of the School of Dentistry since the school opened its doors in 1875. She joined the U-M faculty in 1992 as assistant professor and was promoted through the academic ranks to full professor in 2001. In 2002 she was named the William K. and Mary Anne Najjar professor of periodontics and chair of the Department of Periodontics and Oral Medicine. She chaired the department for 10 years. On September 1, 2013, she began her first five-year term as dean. From the start, McCauley reached out to connect with alumni, faculty, staff, and students "so we can all work together to build on our school's heritage of excellence in education, patient care, research and community outreach," she said.[1]

As deans before her had recognized, it was one thing to have a world-renowned reputation, but it was another thing to keep it. McCauley understood that future success would be dependent on creating systems and technologies designed for organizational effectiveness, restructuring key administrative functions for more efficient operations, and balancing the school's budget for long-term sustainability. It also was clear that the academic health center environment

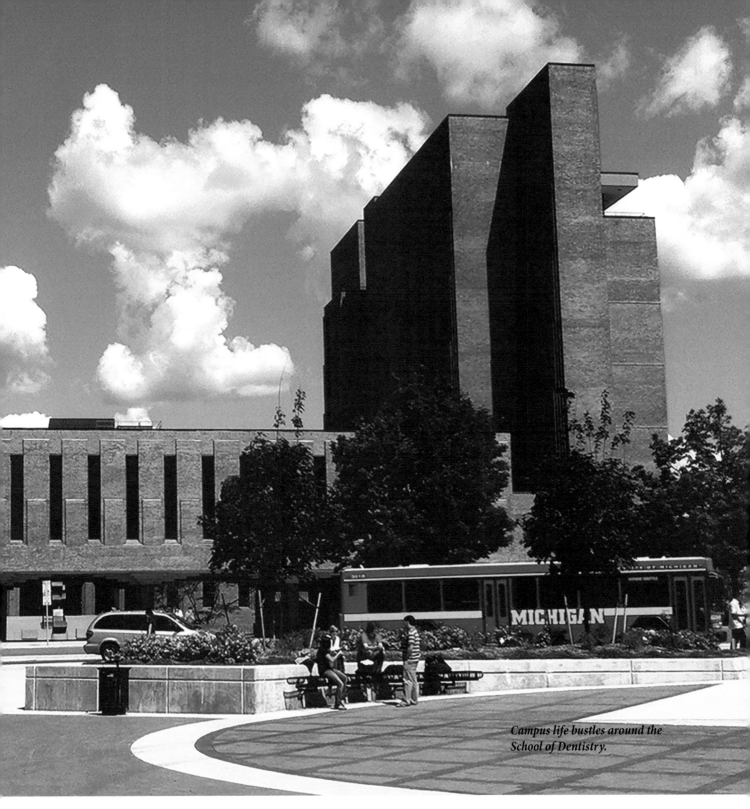

*Campus life bustles around the School of Dentistry.*

was changing rapidly and that the gap between scientific knowledge, education, and patient care was large and expanding. The ability to respond to the changing environment was essential.

## The Strategic Plan

Complacency was not an option and McCauley wasted no time in putting plans in motion. A multidisciplinary team of students, faculty, and staff led by Dr. Lynn Johnson was organized and asked to develop a strategic plan that would lead the school into the future. The team started with an overall vision of building upon the strengths of the university and the state, to enable a diverse University of Michigan School of Dentistry to lead the science and practice of dentistry with preeminent research, contemporary and engaged learning, and exemplary

### The Mission Statement

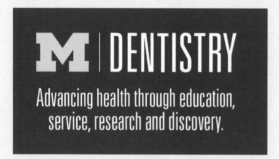

**M | DENTISTRY**

Advancing health through education, service, research and discovery.

### Core Values:

*Compassion:* Encourage a culture of collaboration, collegiality, and helpfulness based on empathy and respect.

*Leadership:* Shape the future leaders of dentistry.

*Excellence:* Be the best at all we do.

*Responsibility:* Expect integrity, professionalism, and accountability to ensure ethical decision-making.

*Trust:* Commit to honest, transparent communication to build relationships.

*Creativity:* Challenge existing knowledge to foster problem-solving and new discovery.

*Inclusion:* Embrace and celebrate our diverse community.

### The Domains:

The five domains were:
- People
- Education
- Research and discovery
- Patient care
- Responsible growth and sustainability

patient care in a vital and sustainable manner. From this vision emerged a simple, yet powerful mission statement driven by seven core values.[2]

As the strategic plan developed, it was organized into five domains, each with its own vision statement. The domains provide the foundation upon which the school sets goals and evaluates processes that define the vision of the strategic plan. The new mission statement, core values, and domains serve as the guiding principles for how the school cares for patients, conducts research, and trains the next generation of leaders, scientists, and clinicians. The strategic plan is a responsive document, subject to rigorous review and based on outcome measures identified, and adapted in response to changes in the environment and results achieved. This plan builds on strengths, informs business decisions, and guides the investments of energy and resources. The strategic plan, when presented to the faculty, received overwhelming support.

## No More Paper Charts

Paper records which had been used for decades to document patient care became a thing of the past when in February 2014, the school ceased using paper records for all new patients. Instead, patient information was recorded, saved, and retrieved electronically via an electronic patient record (EPR). The EPR ensures that all of a patient's information is secure, in one place, and that referring dentists

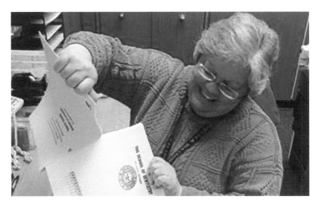

*Administrative Specialist Jean Thompson relishes the task of shredding the paper records in anticipation of the switch to the Electronic Patient Record system.*

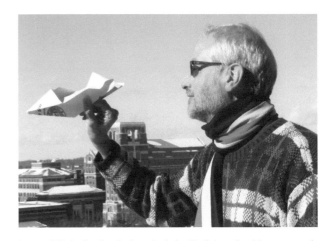

*Dean of Clinics Stephen Stefanac is glad to "jet"-tison the old paper records.*

and physicians can easily provide information to the School of Dentistry providers.[3]

## Interprofessional Education

In early 2015, students from five U-M schools and colleges made academic history. On the and social work studied and worked as teams of professionals.[4,5]

For almost four years, Dr. Carol Anne Murdoch-Kinch, associate dean for Academic Affairs at the School of Dentistry, chaired the U-M Steering Committee for Interprofessional Education. The steering committee was made up of representatives from the College of Pharmacy, the Medical School and Schools of Dentistry, Nursing, Social Work, Public Health, and Kinesiology. The

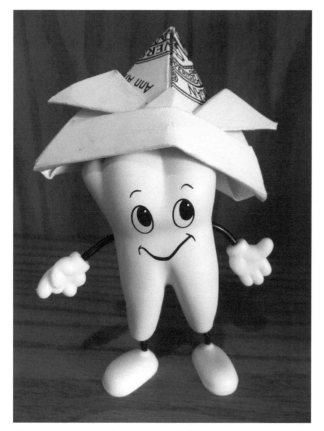

*No more paper records but great material for origami art.*

afternoon of January 14, 52 students gathered in the Kellogg Auditorium to participate in a new course in interprofessional education, Team-Based Clinical Decision Making. The nearly 270 students in dentistry, medicine, nursing, pharmacy,

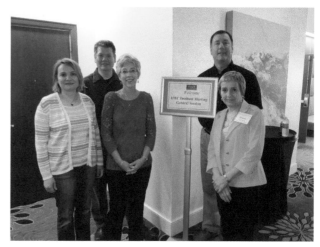

*Representatives of the University of Michigan at the Interprofessional Education Collaborative: (L–R) Maya Hammoud (Medicine), Michael Spencer (Social Work), Carol Anne Murdoch-Kinch (Dentistry, chair), Bruce Mueller (Pharmacy), and Bonnie Hagerty (Nursing).*

interprofessional health education and collaborative care project was designed to break down the traditional silos that separate health professions by creating opportunities for collaborative and engaged learning across disciplines. The committee's hard work culminated in the launch of the U-M Center for Interprofessional Education on July 1, 2015.

**Dr. Carol Anne Murdoch-Kinch** remembers stepping into the Kellogg Auditorium when the class began. Normally, a classroom is a relatively quiet place. An instructor stands before a group of students and talks about a given subject. Students sit, listen, take notes, and ask questions.

But not this time. The interprofessional education class was different. Murdoch-Kinch said:

> What I heard was music to my ears. The classroom was lively. Everyone was participating. Students were talking about their profession and sharing their experiences. Faculty and students were asking questions of each other and exchanging ideas. Everyone was engaged in active learning. I loved it.[6]

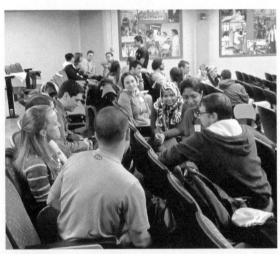

*Students gather in Kellogg Auditorium for one of the university's first courses in interprofessional education and share viewpoints about their profession and their experiences as a health-care professional.*

Case studies were used to enrich active and engaged learning. Applying what they learned, students worked in teams to craft treatment plans for patients with a range of complex health problems.

## Social Media Grows

With the surge of mobile technologies, students, prospective students, faculty, staff, alumni, and parents expect to connect to the school, in one way or the other, with some form a social media.

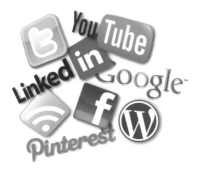

The roots of social media began to take hold with the launch of the school's YouTube and Flickr sites in 2008. A mere handful of YouTube videos grew to more than 1,000 and by the summer of 2014, the school's Flickr photos had received more than a million views. [7,8] A simple Facebook fan page created in 2009 evolved into a Facebook presence that tallied a reach of 1.7 million views in 2016. Social media properties continued to grow with the addition of a student blog in 2010 and a Twitter feed in 2012. LinkedIn and Instagram were added in 2015 and Snapchat in 2017.

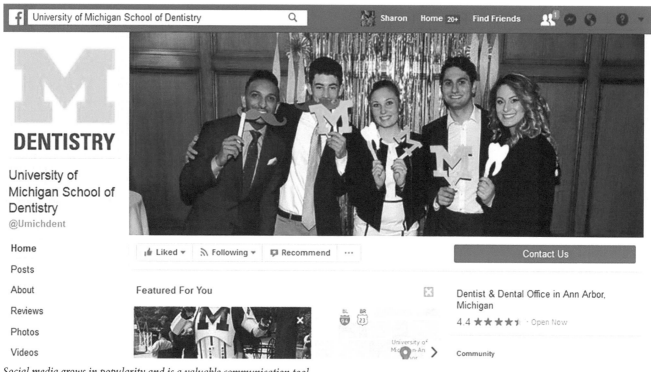

*Social media grows in popularity and is a valuable communication tool.*

## QS World Rankings

In 2015, the School of Dentistry was ranked as the top dental school in the United States and the fourth in the world, according to a survey of institutions of higher learning. *QS World University Rankings*, an annual publication of British Quacquarelli Symonds (QS) Company, has been publishing university rankings since 2010. Rankings were based on academic peer review (40%), faculty/student ratios (20%), faculty citations in research publications (20%), employer reputation (10%), international student ratio to measure the diversity of the student community (5%), and international staff ratio to measure the diversity of the academic staff (5%). While maintaining the #1 ranking in the United States in 2016, the school moved up to the #2 spot worldwide and held both positions in 2017.[9-11]

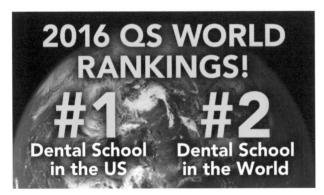

*This image, from the School of Dentistry home page in April 2016, announced the 2016 QS World University Rankings.*

## Accreditation 2016

The school goes through the accreditation process every seven years. It is an enormous undertaking involving every program in the school that

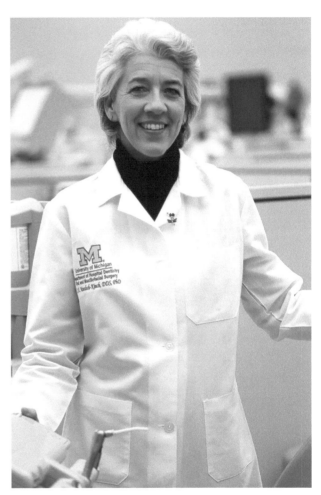

*Dr. Carol Anne Murdoch-Kinch, associate dean for Academic Affairs, guided faculty, staff, and students as they prepared for the important accreditation site visit.*

culminates with a site visit by a team of discipline-specific reviewers from the Commission on Dental Accreditation (CODA). Murdoch-Kinch led the process insuring that the information provided to the review team was both accurate and complete.

At the end of the two-and-a-half-day visit, the CODA site visitors highlighted eight strengths that reflected clear evidence of the school's commitment to its mission, core values, and strategic plan.[12] The school was applauded for the following:

1. Strong leadership team that guides and directs programs and initiatives as well as the staff and faculty's strong commitment to educational excellence.

2. Well-developed and ongoing assessment of student achievement.

3. Innovative curriculum design with an individualized approach, specifically the Pathways program.

4. Commitment of basic science faculty to active self-directed learning opportunities that develop critical thinking and to incorporating clinical correlates into their teaching.

5. Outstanding research funding of the faculty.

6. Solid budget and its transparency as well as strong fund-raising initiatives.

7. Strong community-based clinical educational/outreach program that provides significant benefit to the communities served.

8. Strong alignment with the university in efforts for diversity and inclusion.

Following the site visit, Dean McCauley said in a message to the entire U-M School of Dentistry community:

We've made a strong investment in our curriculum, created a solid budget through careful financial planning and mentored our faculty scientists to elevate our research enterprise. To have our steadfast efforts acknowledged by this esteemed group of our peers is something in which we can take great pride. But we won't stop here. We will continue to advance, innovate and discover and never let go of our commitment to excellence.[13]

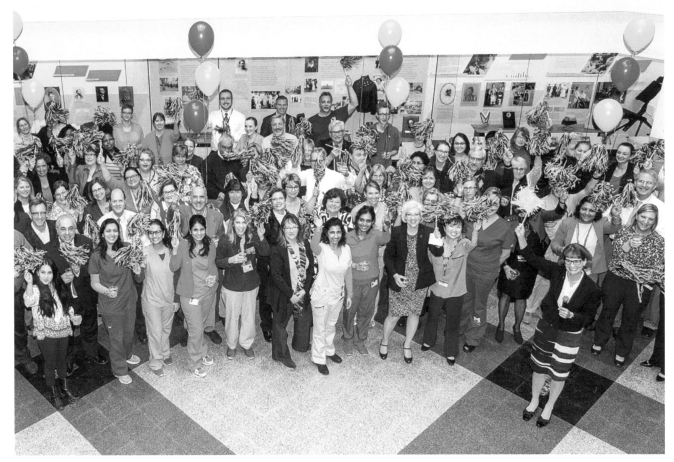

*Faculty, staff, and students gather to celebrate the end of a very positive Commission on Dental Accreditation site visit.*

## Many Voices, Our Michigan

From the very beginning, the School of Dentistry's leadership has been forward-thinking with regard to addressing diversity, equity, and inclusion (DEI), starting with its very first dean—Jonathan Taft. Taft, an early supporter of women dentists, encouraged Miss Ida Gray to apply to the U-M School of Dentistry. Gray who was accepted and graduated in 1890 holds the distinction as the first African American woman in the country to earn a DDS.

A commitment to diversity and inclusion has been further demonstrated over the years. In 1973, Dean William Mann established the Office of Minority Affairs, dedicated to the recruitment of diverse students, staff, and faculty. This office evolved into the Office of Multicultural Affairs in 1999, expanded into the Office of Multicultural Affairs and Recruitment Initiatives in 2008, and then the Office of Diversity and Inclusion since 2014.

The long-standing efforts in this arena, including the Multicultural Audits (1994–1995 and 2006–2007) and the Climate Study (2014–2015), have demonstrated how seriously the school has taken its responsibility to create a climate in which students, staff, faculty, and patients can interact, learn, work, and be treated in a supportive manner.

In September 2015, Schlissel announced that DEI was to be major focus of his presidency and launched a campus-wide initiative to engage all 19 schools and colleges in a DEI strategic planning process. The school, with a solid foundation in place and a renewed commitment to diversity and inclusion in its new strategic plan, whole-heartedly embraced this process.

The campus-wide DEI Strategic Plan, with dentistry's plan (included among the unit plans), was introduced in October 2016. The school's plan, aligned with the university's plan, focuses on dimensions of diversity that include recruitment strategies to maintain a diverse student population as well as strategies for hiring and retaining diverse faculty and staff members. It targets the dental school curriculum and provides intentional educational programing to prepare students to function successfully in a multicultural work environment.

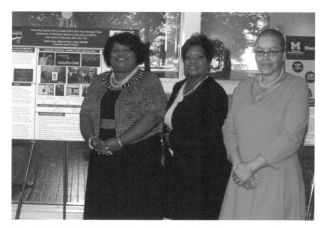

*Katrina Wade-Golden (L), Lead Planning Facilitator in Academic Affairs for the university-wide Diversity, Equity and Inclusion strategic plan, joins School of Dentistry representatives Tina Pryor, human resources director and co-chair of dentistry's diversity plan; and Dinella Crosby, student affairs program specialist in the Office of Diversity and Inclusion.*

Efforts to support DEI through service to our patients is designed to eliminate long-standing disparities in the health status of people of diverse racial, ethnic, and cultural backgrounds with the ultimate goal to improve the quality of services and health outcomes to all School of Dentistry patients.[15]

Institutional climate is also an important part of the plan and is influenced by a host of events planned throughout the year by the Multicultural Affairs Committee (MAC). MAC events promote an understanding of a wide array of cultural variables reflecting difference as well as similarities. In February 2017, the MAC celebrated the 20th anniversary of its founding. Annual activities such as the MLK Day Celebration, Women's History Month

## Alum's portrait of Ida Gray displayed at the president's house

The remarkable journey of Ida Gray continues.

Long celebrated by the School of Dentistry, Gray and her story have gained a wider audience thanks to the artistic talent of an alumnus and the commitment of U-M President Mark Schlissel to further strengthen diversity and inclusion at U-M.

Gray's distinction as the first African American woman in the country to earn a dental degree when she graduated from U-M in 1890 provided historical context for President Schlissel's campus-wide mandate—the Diversity, Equity and Inclusion Strategic Planning Initiative. In launching the five-year plan, Schlissel cited Gray in speeches as an example of the university's significant and often pioneering commitment to diversity in its many forms. Schlissel encouraged schools and colleges to "develop a plan that will be so forward-thinking that a hundred years from now people will still look at it as significant, like the graduation of Dr. Ida Gray."

Gray's higher campus profile didn't end there. A print of the Ida Gray portrait is now displayed prominently at the president's house on South University Avenue. Schlissel's guests from across campus and around the world will encounter the portrait on a wall near the main entrance.

How the portrait made its way to the president's house is a serendipitous tale of Dr. James Lee (DDS 1990), who first thought of creating an artistic gift to honor Gray 25 years ago when he was in dental school. After many years of art instruction and portrait experience, Lee started the pastel portrait of Gray. In September 2015, School of Dentistry administrators were thrilled when he presented the original to the school. When Schlissel learned of the portrait he asked if a print could be made to hang among the many diverse figures in university history displayed in the president's residence.[14]

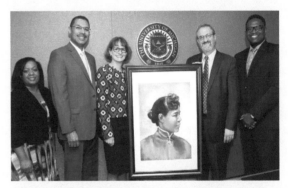

*In March 2016, a delegation from the School of Dentistry presented University of Michigan President Mark Schlissel with a portrait of Dr. Ida Gray. Making the presentation to Schlissel are (L–R) Tina Pryor (human resources director), Dr. James Lee (the artist), Dean Laurie McCauley, President Schlissel, and Dr. Todd Ester (diversity and inclusion director).*

Tea, Taste of Culture (Taste Fest), the Veterans-Day Observance and seminars and monthly "Getting to Know You" brown bag sessions have evolved over the years to promote cultural awareness and esprit de corps in the community.

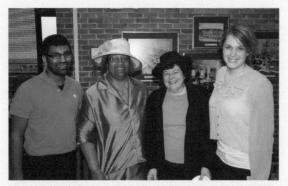

*Big smiles and fun hats were abundant at this Women's Tea event. Enjoying the festivities with the students are Cheryl Quinney, (L, center) and Marita Inglehart (R, center).*

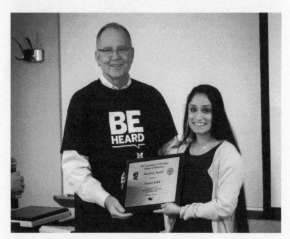

*Henry Temple presents the Ida Gray Award for student leadership to Guneet Kohli (DDS 2017).*

Dean McCauley said:

> It is a core value of our distinguished university and school to assure an excellent, inclusive, and welcoming environment, making the School of Dentistry a great place to work and learn. . . . As a community, we are committed to ensuring diversity in recruiting, selecting, and retaining a diverse and highly engaged workforce.[16]

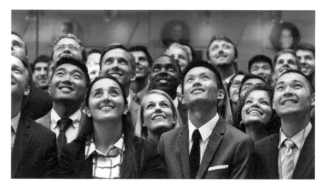

*DDS Class of 2020.*

## Much Needed Renovations and Patience

The wheels of progress often turn slowly and nothing underscores this point more than the request for substantial renovations to the W.K. Kellogg Institute and the Dental Building. A capital project request was first submitted to the university in 2009. Senior Associate Dean Dennis Lopatin and Chief of Staff Erica Hanss presented the Office of the Provost a detailed statement of need, highlighting how the current facilities negatively impact the academic, clinical, and research programs. The request stressed how difficult it would be for the school to maintain its current level of distinction without significant upgrades to these two buildings.

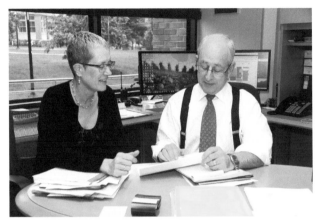

*Chief of Staff Erica Hanss and Senior Associate Dean Dennis Lopatin in the early stages of the capital request planning process.*

This submission was the first step in a multistep process that put dentistry's request on a U-M system-wide list of projects for consideration. Two years later, the school was notified that the Provost's Capital Projects Review Committee had moved the School of Dentistry proposal up the list to the "high priority" category. In a letter to the school from Martha Pollack, vice provost for Academic and Budgetary Affairs, she noted that "projects in the High Priority category will move forward as funding becomes available" with the caveat that it would be "difficult to predict when we

will provide central funding" and that there could be a significant delay before the project could move forward.

In 2013, the university was able to approve funding and the project request was submitted to the governor and state legislature for capital outlay funding consideration in the 2014 budget.[17] It did not move forward in 2014 and 2015, but in June 2016, the Michigan Legislature voted to approve the School of Dentistry request and allocated $30 million in financial support.[18] The following September, the Regents approved the $122 million project that includes a deep renovation of 140,000 square feet (approximately one-third of the existing space) in the W.K. Kellogg Institute and the Dental Building (built in 1940 and 1969, respectively), with the addition of approximately 42,000 square feet.

The long-awaited renovation will create a more welcoming, accessible facility with an improved patient entrance; modern teaching clinics; and open, flexible research space. The architectural firm of SmithGroupJJR was selected to design the project and in April 2017, entered the schematic design phase.[19] The complex process of preparing specifications for a major renovation and addition to the School of Dentistry continues to move forward. The design for this major renovation, projected to cost $140 million, will go to the U-M Board of Regents in March 2018 for final approval.

## Student Entrepreneurs Foster Innovation

In May 2016, three School of Dentistry student-led entrepreneurial projects were featured as part of U-M's Innovate Blue initiative. The Printodontics team developed three-dimensional (3-D) printing software capable of producing a more anatomically accurate artificial tooth with a hardness differential for use in preclinical training. Branden M. Welch (DDS 2018) was the project developer; mentored by Cariology, Restorative Sciences and Endodontics faculty member Dr. Peter Yaman and Professor Emeritus Dr. Joseph Dennison.

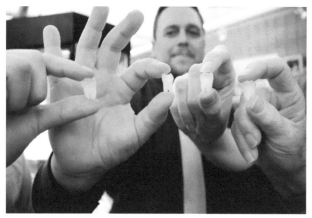

*DDS student entrepreneur, Branden Welch, stands in the background as he and his Printodontics team member hold examples of 3-D printed teeth.*

The Digital Face project was developed by Dr. Ivan Chicchon, a prosthodontics resident in the Class of 2016. The software he developed

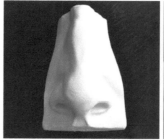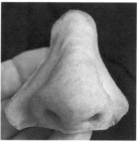

*Software developed by Dr. Ivan Chicchon (MS Pros 2016) was used to create a 3-D model of a nose and to fabricate the custom medical device.*

creates patient-specific 3-D models used in pre-surgical planning for patients requiring facial reconstructive surgery following structural loss from cancer or traumatic injury. The Digital Face program takes imaging data, creates a design proof and delivers the custom device directly to the clinic or hospital.

The third project, Victors Open Arms, featured an important collaboration with Vista Maria, a non-profit organization committed to providing healing and hope to women who have suffered the effects of abuse, neglect, and trauma in Detroit and the greater Michigan area. The student-run, free dental clinic provides much-needed care for traumatized young women and foster care children.

These ventures are prime examples of how the school and the university help students expand their educational experience by nurturing innovative ideas from concept to end product.[20]

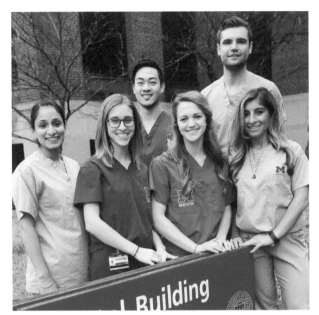

*Victors Open Arms team members from L-R—Guneet Kohli (DDS 2017), Danielle Dunn (DDS 2017), Brian Chang (DDS, 2016), Katherine Johnson (DDS 2017), Bartosz Maska (DDS, 2016) and Jomana Shayota (DDS 2017).*

## Research and Discovery

The U-M School of Dentistry is renowned for its many research accomplishments and talented faculty investigators. The school has long been a place where dynamic thinkers—educators, clinicians, scientists—work diligently to answer tough questions and solve difficult problems to improve care and advance the body of knowledge in dentistry.

Significant research grants and awards are essential to this enterprise. In March 2017, the school-led

interdisciplinary regenerative medicine center, established in 2016, received an $11.7 million award to advance research that integrates engineering and biology, and seeks to regenerate damaged cells, tissues or organs to their full function.

The center, named the Michigan-Pittsburgh-Wyss Resource Center: Supporting Regenerative Medicine in Dental, Oral and Craniofacial Technologies, is led by project directors and principal investigators, Drs. William Giannobile and David Kohn. They will lead a team of scientists from the Medical School, School of Public Health, College of Pharmacy, College of Engineering, the Office of Technology Transfer and the Michigan Institute for Clinical and Health Research. They will also work with other co-investigators from the McGowan Institute at Pittsburgh and the Wyss Institute for Biologically Inspired Engineering at Harvard.[21]

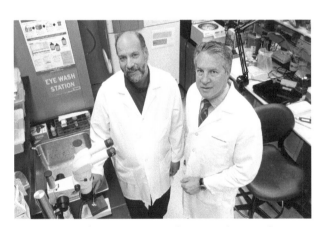

*Regenerative medicine center project directors and principal investigators, Drs. William Giannobile (R) and David Kohn (L).*

Two additional major NIH grants totaling $18.3 million dollars were awarded to the school in September 2017. One grant will expand research into predicting caries risk in young children in low socioeconomic and minority population groups where the disparity in prevalence of caries and access to treatment is greater than in the general population. The second grant will assess the efficacy of a new treatment using silver diamine fluoride (SDF), a non-invasive, inexpensive, and simple alternative for treating cavities in children, particularly those with limited access to regular dental care. Principal investigator Dr. Margherita Fontana will lead a team of U-M researchers in both efforts. Also part of the study are researchers from the University of Iowa, New York University, Indiana University, University of Otago in New Zealand, University of Hong Kong, and University of Baltimore. [22]

Head and neck cancer is the sixth most common cancer in the world with a grim prognosis. In October 2017, Dr. Nisha D'Silva was awarded a $8.1 million Sustaining Outstanding Achievement in Research award, or SOAR, for her continuing research into the molecular pathways that control the spread and recurrence of head and neck cancer. D'Silva and her team will focus their research efforts on invasion because it is a defining feature of head and neck cancer and a key factor in how this cancer spreads. Identifying and understanding the underlying mechanisms that control invasion have the potential to generate new treatment strategies and ultimately improve the survival rates of patients with this lethal form of cancer. The prestigious SOAR grant speaks volumes about how the NIDCR views D'Silva's research track record and her potential moving forward. [23]

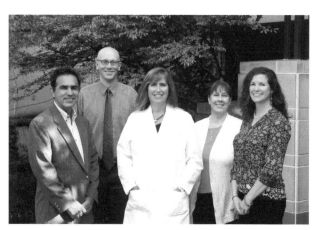

*School of Dentistry researchers who are part of the two new NIH grants include, from left, Dr. Carlos González-Cabezas, Dr. James Boynton, principal investigator Dr. Margherita Fontana, research associate Susan Flannagan, and project manager Emily Yanca.*

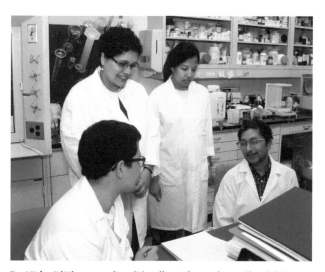

*Dr. Nisha D'Silva , standing (L), talks with members of her lab, from (L), DDS student Tarek Metwally (DDS 2018), Dr. Pruijanka Singh, a research fellow; and Dr. Rajat Banerjee, a research investigator.*

## Caring for Patients with Special Needs

Patients with developmental disabilities, cognitive impairments, blindness or hearing loss, complex medical problems, stress disorders related to military service, or vulnerable conditions unique to the elderly often need special accommodations to receive dental care. A new special needs dental clinic, temporarily located in the Community Dental Center in downtown Ann Arbor, offers patients access to care at a facility with specialized equipment that will allow dentists and dental hygienists to provide care not available at most traditional dental clinics.

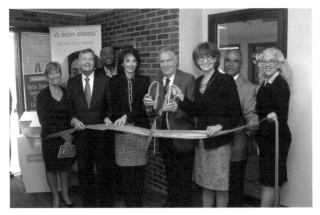

*Participating in the ribbon-cutting ceremony are, from left: Delta Dental Foundation board members Ann Flermoen, James Hallan and Larry Crawford; Teri Battaglieri, Director of the Delta Dental Foundation; board member John Breza; Dean Laurie McCauley, board member Joe Harris; and Dr. Carol Anne Murdoch-Kinch, Associate Dean for Academic Affairs at the dental school.*

The Delta Dental of Michigan Integrated Special Care Clinic was created with the help of a $2 million commitment from the Delta Dental Foundation. The permanent clinic is part of the major School of Dentistry renovation, awaiting Regents approval, expected to be completed in 2022.

Just as important as the physical accommodations are the educational opportunities for dental students and student hygienists. The School of Dentistry is enhancing its curriculum so that students are trained in the best practices for communicating and collaborating with other members of the healthcare team, while treating patients with a wide variety of physical and mental limitations and conditions.

"Immersing our students in new interprofessional integrated care models is the wave of the future for all patients, but it has particular value for special needs patients, and we will lead the way in this area," McCauley stressed. The plan is to implement an integrated collaborative practice model in which multiple health professionals, including dentists and dental hygienists, social workers, behaviorists, physicians, nurses and pharmacists, collaborate to provide optimal comprehensive care for patients with special healthcare needs.[24]

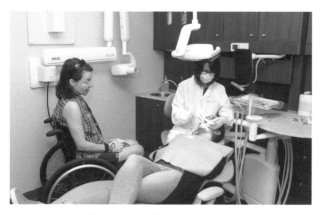

*Diane Kelly, left, talks with dental hygienist Chris Ropp and Manasi Vasavada, a dental student filling the role of patient, during a tour showing the features of the new special needs clinic. Kelly, who has received dental care for 11 years at the Community Dental Center's regular clinic, said the new clinic fills an important need. "I know so many people who will benefit from this," she said.*

## DDS Meets MBA: A New Degree Program

A new joint DDS/MBA degree program was announced in October 2017 by the University of Michigan Ross School of Business. The School of Dentistry put together its proposal for a joint DDS/MBA with the help of three Class of 2019 dental students who saw a growing need for an MBA option in the dental school curriculum. Jae Han, Thomas Paron and Marc Huetter, helped administrators survey interest in the student body and research how other dental schools around the country with joint MBAs have structured their programs. Adding the MBA will extend the normal DDS schedule from four to five years.

> "This is a significant new option for our students that will elevate their leadership capacity and skills," said Dean Laurie McCauley. "The practice

of dentistry, like most health care professions, is in a period of evolution. This program will develop leaders who can advance new practice models that are data-driven and patient-centric. Partnering with the highly-ranked Ross School is a great opportunity for our students."

Jae Young Han is the first dental student to apply to the new program. While he plans to go into private practice, his interests go beyond running a practice. He sees opportunities in many ancillary aspects of dentistry and general health care, such as non-profit service, reducing health care costs, interprofessional education and collaboration, the engineering of surgical tools, practice management, and insurance efficiencies to name few. Whether it is technological advancement, streamlined administration, or insurance reformation, Han sees that he will need the skill set and experience to become an effective, impactful leader in both dentistry and business.[25]

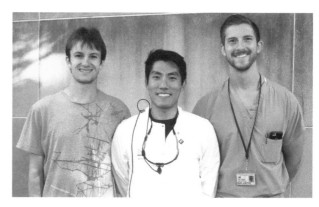

*Jae Young Han, center, enlisted the help of classmates Thomas Paron, (L), and Marc Huetter (R), in putting together a proposal and research promoting a joint DDS-MBA program.*

## Reflections

On February 16, 2017, the U-M Board of Regents approved a second five-year term for Dean McCauley. The reappointment, recommended by Interim Provost Paul Courant, is effective from September 1, 2018, through August 31, 2023.

In announcing the reappointment, Courant called McCauley "an engaged and visible leader." He cited numerous areas of excellence documented during an extensive review for the reappointment. He said McCauley has motivated and guided the school toward the goals in its strategic plan, and led the school through a national dental accreditation process that exceeded expectations in numerous key areas. He said she advocates for diversity and inclusiveness, and works with other health-care deans to promote collaboration among campus units. He noted that the School of Dentistry was at the time ranked No.1 in the country and No. 2 in the world.

"I am confident that she will continue to lead in ways that enhance the school's excellence," Courant said.[26] To that end, it was with great pride that in July 2017 McCauley announced to the school that Shanghai Ranking listed the U-M School of Dentistry No. 1 in Dentistry and Oral Sciences in its Global Ranking of Academic Subjects 2017. The ranking measures research productivity, research quality, extent of international collaboration, amount of research published in top journals, and the number of significant academic awards faculty receive from professional organizations.

Independent reviews like the Shanghai Ranking reflect the school's commitment to being one of the world's leading institutions for dental education and research. "We have a long tradition as leaders in dentistry and rankings like this are one way to gauge our success," McCauley said. "But we know that excellence means always improving, and every day I see our students, faculty and staff focused on finding new and better ways to advance our mission in education,

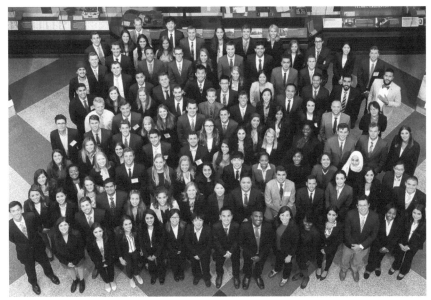

*The journey begins—DDS Class of 2021 look to the future as they pose for their first class photo during orientation on June 26, 2017.*

service, research and discovery. Their commitment is ultimately the best indicator of our success."

As McCauley embarks on her second term, she has emphasized the ongoing challenge for students, faculty, staff and administrators. The school must continue to respect the time-honored traditions that brought it to this place of excellence, yet it must constantly study trends in dentistry and education to ensure that U-M students will be the leaders of the profession moving forward. "It's balancing the excellence, the tradition, and our core values, but reaching out beyond those values to be in a better place, to be contemporary, to be at the leading edge," McCauley said.

It is a commitment to excellence that has been the hallmark of the University of Michigan School of Dentistry for nearly a century and a half.

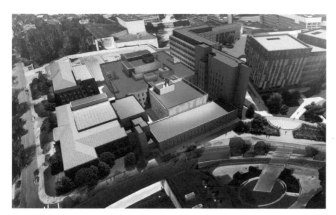 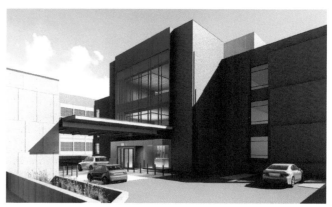

*On March 29, 2018, the U-M Board of Regents approved a schematic design for the $140 million renovation/addition to the School of Dentistry complex. The project will create a more welcoming, accessible facility with an improved patient entrance; modern teaching clinics; and open, flexible research space. The photo on the left shows a three-story addition (highlighted in blue) to be constructed in the central courtyard and a new entrance off the Fletcher parking structure on the north side (right photo).*

# Acknowledgements

As with our rich history, it was the contributions of many people, past and present, that made this work possible. I would like to express my gratitude to all those who contributed to this book, provided support, talked things over, read, wrote, offered comments, allowed me to quote their remarks, and assisted in the editing, proofreading, and design.

I am especially grateful to Dean Laurie McCauley who invited me to see this project through to the end. A huge thank you goes to Jerry Mastey for his work compiling the school's *Encyclopedic Survey—1975–2015* for the bicentennial. Jerry took the *Encyclopedic Survey* and expanded it. His initial draft provided the foundation upon which this work is based.

Writing, fact checking, and going through hundreds of photographs to enrich the School of Dentistry history were essential to this project. I am indebted to those who agreed to be interviewed or provided personal correspondence to enhance the school's history. Special thanks go Henry Kanar, Jack Gobetti, Richard Johnson, Jed Jacobson, Christian Stohler, James McNamara, Emerson Robinson, Charlotte Mistretta, Pat Schultz, John Squires, Karen Ross Peterson, Sandra Sonner Klinesteker, Richard Christiansen, John Drach, Dennis Lopatin, Martha Somerman, Dennis Fasbinder, Lisa Tedesco, Don Heys, Lloyd "Bud" Straffon, Robert Bagramian, Raymond Gist, Marilyn Woolfok, Dan Bruell, Lynn Monson, Vidya Ramaswamy, Carol Ann Murdoch-Kinch, Pattie Katcher, and Lynn Johnson. The Sindecuse Museum of Dentistry staff Shannon O'Dell, Sam Waldron, and Adam Johnson were extremely helpful locating photos, teaching me how to use the image retrieval software, and scanning images, negatives, and other artifacts.

And a very special and heartfelt thanks goes to the School of Dentistry's Chief of Staff Erica Hanss. Erica's institutional knowledge and access to many archived School of Dentistry documents and files were invaluable throughout the process. Equally important were her constant encouragement, support, and feedback.

And to my husband, Stephen Bayne, who kept me grounded and whose sage advice and constant support guided me through this project.

The *Victors for Dentistry (1962–2017)* was prepared for publication to coincide with the University of Michigan Bicentennial Celebration.

Director of Communications....Sharon Grayden

Researcher/Writer....................Sharon Grayden

Researcher/Writer....................Jerry Mastey

Designer....................................Kenneth Rieger

Photographers...........................Keary Campbell, Per Kjeldsen, Jerry Mastey, Lynn Monson, Erica Hanss, Jared Van Ittersum, Celia Alcumbrack-McDaniel, Stephen Stefanac, Sharon Grayden, Stephen Bayne, and the Sindecuse Museum of Dentistry Archives.

The Regents of the University of Michigan (*January 1, 2017–December 31, 2018*)

Michael J. Behm, Mark J. Bernstein, Shauna Ryder Diggs, Denise Ilitch, Andrea Fischer, Andrew C. Richner, Ron Weiser, Katherine E. White, and Mark S. Schlissel (ex officio).

# References

## Chapter 1  The Mann Years (1962–1981)

1. American Council on Education, Commission on the Survey of Dentistry in the United States. 1961. *The Survey of Dentistry: The Final Report.* Washington, DC: American Council on Education.

2. University of Michigan, School of Dentistry. October 1962. *Alumni Bulletin.* Ann Arbor: Bentley Historical Library, University of Michigan.

3. Prospectus for New Building. February 12, 1964. School of Dentistry statements of need. Ann Arbor: Bentley Historical Library, University of Michigan.

4. University of Michigan, School of Dentistry. Winter 1986. *Alumni News,* p. 1.

5. University of Michigan, School of Dentistry. Winter 1986. *Alumni News,* p. 3.

6. University of Michigan, School of Dentistry. 1970. *Alumni Bulletin,* p. 3.

7. Comstock, Frank. ca. 1966. Log of the new dental building from Comstock Notes, SMD0989.0005. Ann Arbor: Sindecuse Museum of Dentistry, University of Michigan.

8. University of Michigan, School of Dentistry. 1968. *Alumni Bulletin,* p. 3.

9. "Workmen at 'U' Unearth Casket and a Mystery Along with It." June 6, 1966. *Ann Arbor News.* Retrieved from http://oldnews.aadl.org/aa_news_19660606-workmen_at_u_unearth_casket.

10. University of Michigan, School of Dentistry. Summer/Fall 1995. *DentalUM,* p. 8.

11. University of Michigan, School of Dentistry. 1971. *Alumni Bulletin,* p. 51.

12. University of Michigan, School of Dentistry. 1970. *Alumni Bulletin,* p. 3.

13. UMichDent. (n.d.). Home. *YouTube Channel.* Retrieved from http://www.youtube.com/user/UMichDent on August 1, 2017.

14. University of Michigan, School of Dentistry. September 1, 1971, *Memo from the Dean,* p. 4.

15. University of Michigan, School of Dentistry. October 22, 1971. *Memo from the Dean,* p. 7.

16. University of Michigan, School of Dentistry (Spring/Summer 2004). *DentalUM,* p. 80.

17. Department of Commerce, U.S. Bureau of the Census, Population Division. 1996 *Population of State and Counties of the United States: 1790–1990.* Retrieved from https://www.census.gov/population/www/documentation/twps0081/twps0081.pdf on August 3, 2017.

18. Michigan, Demographics, Historical Population, U.S. Census Bureau 1910–2010. July 30, 2017. In *Wikipedia, the Free Encyclopedia.* Retrieved from https://en.wikipedia.org/w/index.php?title=Michigan&oldid=793136534 on July 31, 2017.

19. University of Michigan, Office of Capital Planning. April 13, 1973. Meeting minutes. Ann Arbor: Bentley Historical Library, University of Michigan.

20. Long-Range Planning Subcommittee on School and College Planning. December 1, 1972. Summary of the subcommittee's meeting with the School of Dentistry. Ann Arbor: Bentley Historical Library, University of Michigan.

21. University of Michigan, School of Dentistry. October 8, 1979. *Head Count Enrollment—Fall Term.* Document Dean Mann folder. Ann Arbor: Bentley Historical Library, University of Michigan.

22. University of Michigan, School of Dentistry. 1970. *Alumni Bulletin,* p. 3.

23. Nach, Brian J. Summer 1973. "The Comprehensive Health Manpower Training Act of 1971: Panacea or Placebo?" *Catholic University of Law Review,* 22(4): 829–846.

Retrieved from http://scholarship.law.edu/lawreview/vol22/iss4/6.

24. Mann, William R. April 22, 1972. School of Dentistry's Financial Picture. Letter written to Vice President for Academic Affairs, Allan Smith. Ann Arbor: Bentley Historical Library, University of Michigan.

25. Mann, William R. August 3, 1972. Capitation Grant Award. Letter to Vice President for Academic Affairs, Allan Smith. Ann Arbor: Bentley Historical Library, University of Michigan.

26. Congressional Quarterly. 1972. "Health Manpower: $2.9 Billion for Fiscal 1972–1974." *CQ Almanac 1971*, 27th ed., 03-527-03-533. Washington, DC: Congressional Quarterly. Retrieved from http://library.cqpress.com/cqalmanac/cqal71-1253738.

27. Mann, William R. April 13, 1973. School of Dentistry budget meeting. Meeting minutes. Ann Arbor: Bentley Historical Library, University of Michigan.

28. Mann, William R. January 6, 1975. School of Dentistry appropriations and funding. Letter to Vice President of Academic Affairs Frank Rhodes. Ann Arbor: Bentley Historical Library, University of Michigan.

29. Michigan State Legislature. 1975. *Public and Local Acts of the Legislature of the State of Michigan—Regular Session of 1975*. Compiled by Legal Services. Lansing, Michigan: Department of Management and Budget, pp. 1010–1011.

30. University of Michigan, School of Dentistry. 1972. *Alumni Bulletin*, pp. 102–103.

31. University of Michigan, School of Dentistry. 1977–1978. Annual Report to the President of the University. Ann Arbor: Bentley Historical Library, University of Michigan, p. 3.

32. University of Michigan, School of Dentistry. 1972. *Alumni Bulletin*, p. 32.

33. University of Michigan, School of Dentistry. 1973. *Alumni Bulletin*, p. 51.

34. University of Michigan, School of Dentistry. Fall 2006. *DentalUM*, p. 29.

35. University of Michigan, School of Dentistry. March 18, 1970. *SSF Relater, a Publication by and for Students, Staff and Faculty*.

36. University of Michigan, School of Dentistry. Spring/Summer, 2015. *DentalUM*, p. 24.

37. Robinson, Emerson and Bagramian, Robert. "The Community Practice Program at the University of Michigan, Ann Arbor, U.S.A." *Community Dentistry and Oral Epidemiology*, 2: 269–272. doi:10.1111/j.1600–0528.1974.tb01796.x

38. University of Michigan, School of Dentistry. Fall 1978. *Alumni News*, pp. 1–2.

39. University of Michigan, School of Dentistry. 1981–1982. Annual Report to the President of the University. Ann Arbor: Bentley Historical Library, University of Michigan.

40. University of Michigan, School of Dentistry. 1972. *Alumni Bulletin*, p. 118.

41. University of Michigan, School of Dentistry. 1972. *Alumni Bulletin*, p. 119.

42. University of Michigan, School of Dentistry. 1970. *Alumni Bulletin*, p. 25.

43. University of Michigan, School of Dentistry. 1975–1976. *Alumni Bulletin*, p. 22.

44. University of Michigan, School of Dentistry. 1977–1978. Annual Report to the President of the University. Ann Arbor: Bentley Historical Library, University of Michigan.

45. University of Michigan, School of Dentistry. Fall 1980. *Alumni News*, p. 4.

46. University of Michigan, School of Dentistry. Summer/Fall 1997. *DentalUM*, p. 32.

47. University of Michigan, School of Dentistry. January/February 1979. *Michigan Dental Explorer*, p. 3.

48. University of Michigan, School of Dentistry. 1970. *Alumni Bulletin*, p. 18.
49. University of Michigan, School of Dentistry. Fall 1979. *Alumni News*, p. 1.
50. University of Michigan, School of Dentistry. 1970. *Alumni Bulletin*, p. 59.
51. University of Michigan, School of Dentistry. Spring/Summer 2002. *DentalUM*, p. 34.

## Chapter 2  The Doerr Years (1981–1982)

1. University of Michigan, School of Dentistry. Summer 1981. *Alumni News*, p.1.
2. University of Michigan, School of Dentistry. 1977–1978. Annual Report to the President of the University. Ann Arbor: Bentley Historical Library, University of Michigan.
3. University of Michigan, School of Dentistry. 1978–1979. Annual Report to the President of the University. Ann Arbor: Bentley Historical Library, University of Michigan.
4. University of Michigan, School of Dentistry. 1972. *Alumni Bulletin*, p. 100.
5. University of Michigan, School of Dentistry. Spring 1982. *Alumni Bulletin*, pp. 1–2.
6. University of Michigan, School of Dentistry. 1980–1985. Tuition Reports. Ann Arbor: School of Dentistry's Office of Academic Affairs.
7. University of Michigan, School of Dentistry. Fall 1980. *Alumni News*, p. 1.
8. University of Michigan, School of Dentistry. Summer 1981. *Alumni News*, p. 8.
9. University of Michigan, School of Dentistry. Spring 1982. *Alumni News*, p. 4.
10. University of Michigan, School of Dentistry. October 1990. *Alumni News Supplement*, p. 3.
11. Faculty History Project. 2011. Memoir: Robert Edward Doerr. Regent's Proceedings 966. Retrieved from http://um2017.org/faculty-history/faculty/robert-edward-doerr/memoir on August 9, 2017.

## Chapter 3  The Christiansen Years (1982–1987)

1. University of Michigan, School of Dentistry. Summer 1981. *Alumni News*, p. 1.
2. University of Michigan, School of Dentistry. 1981–1982. University of Michigan Instructional Salary Comparison by Department. Ann Arbor: Bentley Historical Library, University of Michigan.
3. University of Michigan, School of Dentistry. 1983–1984. Annual Report to the President of the University. Ann Arbor: Bentley Historical Library, University of Michigan.
4. Christiansen, Richard L. July 2, 1984. Memo to Budget Priorities Committee Chairman Dr. Fred Burgett. Ann Arbor: Bentley Historical Library, University of Michigan.
5. University of Michigan, School of Dentistry. 1984–1985. Annual Report to the President of the University. Ann Arbor: Bentley Historical Library, University of Michigan.
6. University of Michigan, School of Dentistry. 1985–1986. Annual Report to the President of the University. Ann Arbor: Bentley Historical Library, University of Michigan.
7. University of Michigan, School of Dentistry. 1986–1987. Annual Report to the President of the University. Ann Arbor: Bentley Historical Library, University of Michigan.
8. University of Michigan, School of Dentistry. 1982–1987. Admissions records. Ann Arbor: School of Dentistry's Office of Admissions.

9. University of Michigan, School of Dentistry. Fall 2004. *DentalUM*, p. 34.

10. University of Michigan, School of Dentistry. Fall 1984. *Alumni News*, p. 5.

11. University of Michigan, School of Dentistry. Spring 1998. *DentalUM*, p. 4.

12. University of Michigan, School of Dentistry. Fall 1986. *Alumni News*, pp 8–9.

13. University of Michigan, School of Dentistry. Winter 1986. *Alumni News*, p. 12.

14. University of Michigan, School of Dentistry. Fall 1982. *Alumni News*, p. 1.

15. McNamara, James. (n.d.). Founding Director, Robert J. Moyers. Retrieved from http://chgd.umich.edu/about/50th-anniversary/founding-director-robert-e-moyers/ on August 10, 2017.

16. University of Michigan, School of Dentistry. Fall 1984. *Alumni News*, p. 1.

17. University of Michigan, School of Dentistry. Fall 1986. *Alumni News*, p. 11.

18. Christiansen, Richard. 1987. Christiansen Correspondence, Box 26. *School of Dentistry (University of Michigan) Records: 1873–2010*. Ann Arbor: Bentley Historical Library, University of Michigan.

## Chapter 4   The Kotowicz Years (1987–1989)

1. Duderstadt, James. March 27, 1987. Memo to School of Dentistry faculty from the provost and vice president for Academic Affairs. Ann Arbor: Bentley Historical Library, University of Michigan.

2. University of Michigan, School of Dentistry. Fall 2002. *DentalUM*, p. 6.

3. University of Michigan, School of Dentistry. Fall 1988. "From the Dean," *Alumni News*, p. 5.

4. University of Michigan, School of Dentistry. Fall/Winter 1987–1988. *Alumni News*, p. 1.

5. University of Michigan, School of Dentistry. Spring/Summer 2002. *DentalUM*, p. 6.

6. University of Michigan, School of Dentistry. Winter 1990–1991. *DentalUM*, pp. 6–9.

7. University of Michigan, School of Dentistry. Fall 1988. "Dean's Message," *Alumni News*, p. 5.

8. University of Michigan, School of Dentistry. Winter 1990–1991. *DentalUM*, pp 6–9.

9. University of Michigan, School of Dentistry. Fall/Winter 1987–88. "Research Duel with OSU; A Great New Tradition Begins!" *Alumni News*, p. 10.

10. University of Michigan, School of Dentistry. December 1, 1972. Summary of the meeting of the Long-Range Planning Subcommittee on School and College Planning with the School of Dentistry (Document). Ann Arbor: Bentley Historical Library, University of Michigan.

11. University of Michigan, School of Dentistry. 1972. *Alumni Bulletin*, p. 34.

12. University of Michigan, School of Dentistry. July 1989. *Alumni News Supplement*, p. 2.

## Chapter 5   The Machen Years (1989–1995)

1. University of Michigan, School of Dentistry. Fall/Winter 1989–1990. *Alumni News*, p. 1.

2. Machen, J. Bernard. October 23, 1989. Dean Machen's address to the School of Dentistry faculty (Document). Ann Arbor: Bentley Historical Library, University of Michigan.

3. University of Michigan, School of Dentistry. Fall/Winter 1989–1990. *Alumni News*, p. 4.

4. Faculty History Project. 2011 Memoir: Dennis F. Turner, Regents' Proceedings 85. Retrieved from http://um2017.org/faculty-history/faculty/dennis-f-turner/memoir on August 17, 2017.

5. University of Michigan, School of Dentistry. December 1991. *DentalUM Supplement*, p. 8.

6. University of Michigan, School of Dentistry. 1978–1979. Annual Report to the President of the University. Ann Arbor: Bentley Historical Library, University of Michigan, p. 3.

7. University of Michigan, School of Dentistry. Summer 1990. *Alumni News*, p. 8.

8. University of Michigan, School of Dentistry. Fall 2002. *DentalUM*, p. 21.

9. University of Michigan, School of Dentistry. March 1991. *DentalUM Supplement*, p. 7.

10. Faculty History Project. 2011 Memoir: Lysle E. Johnston, Jr., Regents' Proceedings 26. Retrieved from http://um2017.org/faculty-history/faculty/lysle-e-johnston-jr/memoir on August 9, 2017.

11. University of Michigan, School of Dentistry. October 1990. *Alumni News Supplement*, p. 2.

12. University of Michigan, School of Dentistry. 1999–2001. *University of Michigan Bulletin*. Ann Arbor: Bentley Historical Library, University of Michigan, pp. 155–156.

13. University of Michigan, School of Dentistry. Fall 2000. *DentalUM*, p. 33.

14. University of Michigan, School of Dentistry. Winter 1992. *DentalUM*, p. 18.

15. University of Michigan, School of Dentistry. Fall 1999. *DentalUM*, pp. 42–45.

16. University of Michigan, School of Dentistry. Fall 1991. *DentalUM*, pp. 6–8.

17. University of Michigan, School of Dentistry. 1993. Minutes of the September 23, 1993, School of Dentistry faculty meeting. Ann Arbor: Bentley Historical Library, University of Michigan.

18. University of Michigan, School of Dentistry. Spring 1994. *DentalUM*, p. 6.

19. University of Michigan, School of Dentistry. Spring/Summer 2005. *DentalUM*, p. 31.

20. University of Michigan, School of Dentistry. Spring/Summer 2005. *DentalUM*, p. 35.

21. University of Michigan, School of Dentistry. "Roy and Natalie Roberts Making Donor History with a $10 Million Gift Commitment." Spring 1998. *DentalUM Special Edition*, Report on the Campaign for Michigan,

22. University of Michigan, School of Dentistry. Fall 1991. *DentalUM*, p. 12.

23. University of Michigan, School of Dentistry. Winter 1992. *DentalUM*, p. 3.

24. University of Michigan, School of Dentistry. Winter 1995–1996). *DentalUM*, p. 12.

25. University of Michigan, School of Dentistry. Summer/Fall 1995. *DentalUM*, p. 12.

26. University of Michigan, School of Dentistry. Summer/Fall 1995. Letter from the Dean. *DentalUM*, p. 2.

## Chapter 6   The Kotowicz Years (1995–2003)

1. University of Michigan, School of Dentistry. Fall 2002. *DentalUM*, pp. 21–22.

2. University of Michigan, School of Dentistry. Summer/Fall 1997. "From the Dean." *DentalUM*, IFC.

3. University of Michigan, School of Dentistry. Fall 2002. *DentalUM*, pp. 23–24.

4. University of Michigan, School of Dentistry. Fall 2002. *DentalUM*, p. 28.

5. University of Michigan, School of Dentistry. Summer/Fall 1995. *DentalUM*, p. 17.

6. University of Michigan, School of Dentistry. Fall/Winter 1996–1997. *DentalUM*, p. 8.

7. University of Michigan, School of Dentistry. Fall/Winter 1996–1997. *DentalUM*, p. 15.

8. University of Michigan, School of Dentistry. Spring/Summer 2008. *DentalUM*, p. 63.

9. University of Michigan, School of Dentistry. Fall/Winter 1996–1997. *DentalUM*, p. 10.

10. University of Michigan, School of Dentistry. Spring 1980. *Alumni News*, p. 3.

11. University of Michigan, School of Dentistry. Fall 2000. *DentalUM*, p. 9.

12. University of Michigan, School of Dentistry. 1975. *Alumni Bulletin* (Centennial Issue), p. 21.

13. University of Michigan, School of Dentistry. September 8, 2000. 125th anniversary and renovated facilities. Special Moments. Ann Arbor: Bentley Historical Library, University of Michigan.

14. Sindecuse Museum of Dentistry. (n.d.). Danovich Mural. Ann Arbor: Bentley Historical Library, University of Michigan. Retrieved from http://dent.umich.edu/about-school/sindecuse-museum/danovich-mural on August 9, 2017.

15. University of Michigan, School of Dentistry. Fall 2000. *DentalUM*, pp.1, 4–13.

16. University of Michigan, School of Dentistry. Spring/Summer 2004. *DentalUM*, p. 40.

17. University of Michigan, School of Dentistry. Spring/Summer 2005. *DentalUM*, p. 35.

18. University of Michigan, School of Dentistry. Spring/Summer 2005. *DentalUM*, p. 34.

19. University of Michigan, School of Dentistry. Spring/Summer 2005. *DentalUM*, p. 37.

20. University of Michigan, School of Dentistry. Spring 1995. *DentalUM*, p. 9.

21. University of Michigan, School of Dentistry. Summer/Fall 1995. *DentalUM*, p. 18.

22. University of Michigan, School of Dentistry. Spring 1998. *DentalUM*, p. 14.

23. University of Michigan, School of Dentistry. Spring/Summer 2001. *DentalUM*, pp. 5–7.

24. University of Michigan, School of Dentistry. Fall 1999. *DentalUM*, pp. 4–5.

25. University of Michigan, School of Dentistry. Spring/Summer 2000. *DentalUM*, p. 6.

26. University of Michigan, School of Dentistry. Winter 1992. Lysle Johnston Department Update, *DentalUM*, pp. 6–8.

27. University of Michigan, School of Dentistry. Spring/Summer 2000. *DentalUM*, p. 13.

28. University of Michigan, School of Dentistry. (Spring/Summer 2000). *DentalUM*, pp. 12–35.

29. University of Michigan, School of Dentistry. Fall 2000. *DentalUM*, p. 51.

30. University of Michigan, School of Dentistry. Fall 2001 *DentalUM*, p. 43.

31. University of Michigan, School of Dentistry. Spring/Summer 2002. *DentalUM*, pp. 1, 6–8.

## Chapter 7 The Polverini Years (2003–2013)

1. University of Michigan, Board of Regents. 2002–2003. *Proceedings of the Board of Regents*, pp 229–230. Retrieved from https://quod.lib.umich.edu/u/umregproc/ACW7513.2002.001/230?rgn=full+text;view=pdf;q1=Polverini.

2. University of Michigan, School of Dentistry. Fall 2003. *DentalUM*, p. 7.

3. University of Michigan, School of Dentistry. Fall 2005. *DentalUM*, pp. 4–5.

4. University of Michigan, School of Dentistry. Spring/Summer 2004. *DentalUM*, pp.11–14.

5. Bierma, Nathan. December 28, 2005. "'Podcast' Is Lexicon's Word of the Year." *Chicago Tribune*. Special to the Tribune. Retrieved from http://articles.chicagotribune.com/2005-12-28/features/0512270256_1_podcast-new-oxford-american-dictionary-word-origins on August 15, 2017.

6. University of Michigan, School of Dentistry. Fall 2005. *DentalUM*, pp. 10–11.

7. University of Michigan, School of Dentistry. Fall 2007. *DentalUM*, p. 75.

8. University of Michigan, School of Dentistry. March 28, 2017. *School of Dentistry Facts & Figures* (Fact sheet). Ann Arbor: Bentley Historical Library, University of Michigan.

9. Wiernik, J. July 30, 1991. "Dentistry Pioneer Ostrander Dies." *Ann Arbor News*. p. C3.

10. University of Michigan, School of Dentistry. Fall/Winter 2012–2013). *DentalUM*, p. 5.

11. University of Michigan, School of Dentistry. Fall 2007. *DentalUM*, p. 51.

12. University of Michigan, School of Dentistry. Spring/Summer 2008. *DentalUM*, p.63.

13. University of Michigan, School of Dentistry. Spring/Summer 2012. *DentalUM*, p. 28.

14. University of Michigan, School of Dentistry. Fall 2008. *DentalUM*, p. 5.

15. University of Michigan, School of Dentistry. Fall 2009. *DentalUM*, p. 2.

16. University of Michigan, School of Dentistry. Fall/Winter 2013–2014). *DentalUM*, pp. 10–11.

17. University of Michigan, School of Dentistry. Spring/Summer 2013. *DentalUM*, p. 2.

18. University of Michigan, School of Dentistry. 2015. *Polverini Named Distinguished University Professor* (Press release). Retrieved from http://www.dent.umich.edu/news/2015/05/21/polverini-named-distinguished-university-professor.

## Chapter 8  The McCauley Years (2013–2023)

1. University of Michigan, School of Dentistry. Fall/Winter 2013–2014. *DentalUM*, pp. 3–5.

2. University of Michigan, School of Dentistry. *Michigan Dentistry: Leading the Future, Spring 2014 Strategic Plan*. Retrieved from http://media.dent.umich.edu/planning/files/StrategicPlan2014.pdf on August 10, 2017.

3. University of Michigan, School of Dentistry. Spring/Summer 2014. *DentalUM*, p. 14.

4. University of Michigan, School of Dentistry. 2015. *Interprofessional Education Begins at Michigan* (Press release). Retrieved from http://www.dent.umich.edu/news/2015/01/22/interprofessional-education-begins-michigan.

5. University of Michigan, School of Dentistry. Spring/Summer 2015. *DentalUM*, pp. 6–7.

6. University of Michigan, School of Dentistry. Spring/Summer 2015. *DentalUM*, p. 2.

7. University of Michigan, School of Dentistry. 2014. *Milestone: 1 Million+ Flickr Photo Views* (Press release). Retrieved from http://www.dent.umich.edu/news/2014/08/20/milestone-1-million-flickr-photo-views.

8. University of Michigan, School of Dentistry. Fall/Winter 2014–2015. *DentalUM*, p. 6.

9. *QS World University Rankings by Subject 2015—Dentistry*. 2015. Retrieved from https://www.topuniversities.com/university-rankings/university-subject-rankings/2015/dentistry.

10. *QS World University Rankings by Subject 2016—Dentistry*. 2016. Retrieved from https://www.topuniversities.com/university-rankings/university-subject-rankings/2016/dentistry.

11. *QS World University Rankings by Subject 2017—Dentistry*. 2017. Retrieved from https://www.topuniversities.com/university-rankings/university-subject-rankings/2017/dentistry.

12. University of Michigan, School of Dentistry. Spring/Summer 2016. *DentalUM*, p. 11.

13. University of Michigan, School of Dentistry. Spring/Summer 2016. *DentalUM*, *Dean's Message*.

14. University of Michigan, School of Dentistry. Fall/Winter 2016–2017. *DentalUM*, p. 8.

15. University of Michigan, School of Dentistry. May 25, 2016. *Diversity Equity and Inclusion Five Year Strategic Plan*. Retrieved from http://media.dent.umich.edu/publications/UMSD-DEI-multicultural.pdf on August 10, 2017.

16. University of Michigan, School of Dentistry. May 25, 2016. *Diversity, Equity and Inclusion Five Year Strategic Plan, p.6*. Retrieved from http://media.dent.umich.edu/publications/UMSD-DEI-multicultural.pdf on August 10, 2017.

17. Broekhuizen, K. December 19, 2013. "Ann Arbor, Dearborn Campuses Ask State for Capital Outlay Funds." *The University Record*. Retrieved from https://record.umich.edu/articles/ann-arbor-dearborn-campuses-submit-capital-outlay-requests-state.

18. Broekhuizen, Kim. June 9, 2016. "University Projects Approved for Capital Outlay Funding." *The University Record*. Retrieved from https://record.umich.edu/articles/university-projects-approved-capital-outlay-funding.

19. Fitzgerald, Rick. September 15, 2016. "Major Renovation Planned for School of Dentistry." *The University Record*. Retrieved from https://record.umich.edu/articles/major-renovation-planned-school-dentistry.

20. University of Michigan, May 26, 2016. "Dentistry Entrepreneurial Projects Featured by U-M's Innovate Blue Initiative." Retrieved from http://dent.umich.edu/news/2016/05/26/dentistry-entrepreneurial-projects-featured-u-ms-innovate-blue-initiative on June 3, 2016.

21. University of Michigan, School of Dentistry. March 7, 2017. "School of Dentistry Leads Major New Regenerative Medicine Center Funded by NIH." Retrieved from http://www.dent.umich.edu/news/2017/03/07/school-dentistry-leads-major-new-regenerative-medicine-center-funded-nih on October 18, 2017.

22. University of Michigan, School of Dentistry. September 22, 2017. "Two Major NIH Grants to Further Research into Childhood Caries." Retrieved from http://www.dent.umich.edu/news/2017/09/22/two-major-nih-grants-further-research-childhood-caries on October 18, 2017.

23. University of Michigan, School of Dentistry. October 4, 2017. "Dentistry Professor Receives Major NIH Mid-career Grant." Retrieved from http://www.dent.umich.edu/news/2017/10/03/dentistry-professor-receives-major-nih-mid-career-grant on October 18, 2017.

24. University of Michigan, School of Dentistry. October 12, 2017. "Special Needs Dental Clinic Project Moves Forward." Retrieved from http://www.dent.umich.edu/news/2017/10/11/special-needs-dental-clinic-project-moves-forward on October 18, 2017.

25. University of Michigan, School of Dentistry. October 10, 2017. "DDS Meets MBA: New Degree Program Announced." Retrieved from http://www.dent.umich.edu/news/2017/10/11/special-needs-dental-clinic-project-moves-forward on October 18, 2017.

26. University of Michigan, School of Dentistry. February 16, 2017. *U-M Regents Reappoint Dean Laurie McCauley*. Retrieved from http://www.dent.umich.edu/news/2017/02/16/u-m-regents-reappoint-dean-laurie-mccauley on February 16, 2017.

# About the Editor/Author

Sharon Grayden's career in dentistry has spanned four decades. She has been involved in the dental profession as an educator, researcher and administrator; affiliated with three of the best dental schools in the country—the University of Minnesota, University of North Carolina at Chapel Hill and the University of Michigan.

While at the University of Minnesota her career focus began to shift from teaching and research into the communications and public relations arenas. When she joined UNC-Chapel Hill she directed the public relations activities for the dental school that included managing and marketing the continuing education programs and writing and editing the *North Carolina Dental Review*. She joined the University of Michigan School of Dentistry in 2006 and was named director of communications in 2008. In this role she served as the public relations liaison for the school. She generated press releases and public relations pieces, wrote and edited speeches, and served as editor in chief of the school's premier publication, *DentalUM*. She retired from dentistry in 2016 but still remains actively involved with a number of writing, editing and graphic design projects.

# Appendix A
## University of Michigan School of Dentistry Deans (1975–2017)

| | |
|---|---|
| 1875–1903: | Jonathan Taft |
| 1903–1906: | Cyrenus G. Darling (acting) |
| 1907 | Willoughby D. Miller[a] |
| 1907–1916: | Nelville S. Hoff |
| 1916–1934: | Marcus L. Ward |
| 1934–1935: | Chalmers J. Lyons |
| 1935–1950: | Russell W. Bunting |
| 1950–1962: | Paul H. Jeserich |
| 1962–1981: | William R. Mann |
| 1981–1982: | Robert E. Doerr (interim) |
| 1982–1987: | Richard L. Christiansen |
| 1987–1989: | William E. Kotowicz (interim) |
| 1989–1995: | J. Bernard Machen |
| 1995–2002: | William E. Kotowicz |
| 2003–2013: | Peter J. Polverini |
| 2013–present: | Laurie K. McCauley |

a  In 1906, the Board of Regents appointed world-renowned dental educator and scientist Willoughby D. Miller as dean of the University of Michigan School of Dentistry. His term was to begin in the fall of 1907. Dean designee Miller visited Ann Arbor for a few days during the summer prior to assuming the deanship. He then traveled to Ohio to visit relatives and fell ill with appendicitis. He died in Newark, Ohio, on July 27, 1907.

# Appendix B
## Professorships, School of Dentistry, University of Michigan

*ENDOWED PROFESSORSHIPS*

**Robert W. Browne Endowed Professorship**  (established: 2/1/1985)

Lysle E. Johnston, Jr. (1991–2004)
R. Scott Conley (2011–2016)

**William K. and Mary Anne Najjar Endowed Professorship in Dentistry** (established: 2/1/1985)

Martha Somerman (1991–2003)
William V. Giannobile (2003-)

**Drs. Thomas M. and Doris Graber Endowed Professorship in Dentistry** (established: 7/1/1998)

James A. McNamara (1998–2014)
Sunil D. Kapila (2014–2016)

**Robert W. Browne Professorship in Orthodontics** (established: 2/1/2002)

Sunil D. Kapila (2004–2014)

**William K. and Mary Anne Najjar Endowed Professorship in Periodontics** (established: 2/1/2002)

Laurie K. McCauley (2002-)

**Dr. Roy H. Roberts Professorship in Dentistry** (established: 2/1/2002)

Christian S. Stohler (2002)
William E. Kotowicz (2004–2005)
Paul H. Krebsbach (2005–2016)

**Chalmers J. Lyons Endowed Professorship** (established: 9/1/2007)

Joseph I. Helman (2008-)

**Dr. Walter H. Swartz Professorship in Integrated Special Care Dentistry** (established: 2/1/2015)

Carol Anne Murdoch-Kinch (2017-)

**James Hayward Endowed Clinical Professorship in Dentistry** (established: 8/1/2016)

Sean Edwards (2016-)

*COLLEGIATE PROFESSORSHIPS*

**Donald A. Kerr Endowed Collegiate Professorship in Dentistry** (established: 10/1/1997)

Peter J. Polverini (1997)
Thomas E. Carey (2002–2007)
Jacques E. Nor (2011-)

**Richard H. Kingery Endowed Collegiate Professorship in Dentistry** (established: 10/1/1998)

Cun-Yu Wang (2004–2007)
Peter Ma (2009-)

**Samuel D. Harris Collegiate Professorship in Dentistry** (established: 1/1/2000)

Robert J. Feigal (2000–2003)
Jan C.C. Hu (2005-)

**Donald A. Kerr Endowed Collegiate Professorship in Oral Pathology** (established: 2/1/2002)

Paul H. Krebsbach (2002–2005)
Nisha D'Silva (2007-)

**Collegiate Professorship in Periodontics** (established: 12/1/2006)

Hom-Lay Wang (2007-)

**James E. Harris Collegiate Professorship in Orthodontics** (established: 10/1/2008)

Unassigned

**Major M. Ash Collegiate Professorship in Periodontics** (established: 1/1/2011)

Russell Taichman (2011-)

**Lysle E. Johnston, Jr. Collegiate Professorship in Orthodontics** (established: 8/1/2015)

Nan Hatch (2015-)

**Richard Christiansen Collegiate Professorship in Oral and Craniofacial Global Initiatives** (established: 10/1/2015)

Carlos Gonzalez-Cabesas (2015-)

## *UNENDOWED COLLEGIATE PROFESSORSHIPS*

**Marcus L. Ward Professorship of Dentistry** (established: 6/21/1974)

Albert G. Richards (1974–1980)
Major Ash (1984–1989)
Robert G. Craig (1990–1993)
Richard E. Corpron (1993–1996)
Walter E. Loesche (1996–2000)
Joseph Dennison (2001–2005)
Stephen C. Bayne (2011–2016)
Renny Franceschi (2016-)

**William R. Mann Professorship of Dentistry** (established: 9/1/1994)

Nathaniel H. Rowe, Jr. (1994–1997)
Christian S. Stohler (1997–2002)
Charlotte M. Mistretta (2003-)

## *DISTINGUISHED UNIVERSITY PROFESSORSHIPS*

**Jonathan Taft Distinguished University Professor**

Peter J. Polverini (2015)

**Note:** School of Dentistry professorships are traditionaly 5-year, renewable appointments. The duration of the Distinguished University Professorship appointment is unlimited and the title may be retained after retirement.

# Appendix C

## Leaders and Best

### University of Michigan School of Dentistry

#### Past Presidents

##### American Dental Association

1959–1960: Paul H. Jeresich—Ann Arbor (DDS 1924, Dean 1950–1962)

1967–1968: Floyd. D. Ostrander—Ann Arbor (DDS 1934, MS 1940)

2003–2004: Raymond F. Gist—Grand Blanc (DDS 1966)

#### Past Presidents

##### Michigan Dental Association

**1876: University of Michigan School of Dentistry awards first dental degrees.**

1873–1874: D. Claude Hawxhurst[a]—Battle Creek (DDS 1876)

1875–1876: John W. Finch[a]—Adrian (DDS 1879, Honorary)

1883–1884: William H. Dorrence[a]—Ann Arbor (DDS 1879)

1902–1903: E. Alan Honey—Kalamazoo (DDS 1890)

1904–1905: Frederick H. Essig—Dowagiac (DDS 1888)

1908–1909: James W. Lyons—Jackson (DDS 1885)

1912–1913: Marcus L. Ward—Ann Arbor (DDS 1902, DDSc 1905)

1918–1919: Chalmers J. Lyons—Ann Arbor (DDS 1898, DDSc 1911)

1920–1921: Clare G. Bates—Durand (DDS 1897)

1921–1922: Russell W. Bunting—Ann Arbor (DDS 1902, DDSc 1908, Dean 1937–1950)

1924–1925: W.W. Gibson—Grand Rapids (DDS 1915)

1926–1927: J.D. Locke—Grand Rapids (DDS 1918)

1927–1928: William E. Brown—Benton Harbor (DDS 1913)

1928–1929: Percival C. Lowery—Detroit (DDS 1910, Honorary Degree ScD 1940)

1935–1936: Harry F. Parks—Jackson (DDS 1908)

1936–1937: William F. Northrup—Detroit (DDS 1911)

1937–1938: U. Garfield Rickert—Ann Arbor (DDS 1916)

1938–1939: J. Orton Goodsell—Saginaw (DDS 1918)

1939–1940: Paul H. Jeserich—Watervliet (DDS 1924, Dean 1950–1962)

1940–1941: Frederick J. Henry—Grand Rapids (DDS 1918)

1941–1942: Clarence J. Wright—Lansing (DDS 1916)

1942–1943: Lewis E. Hooper—Grosse lle (DDS 1919)

1943–1944: Oliver C. Applegate—Ann Arbor (DDS 1917, DDSc 1937)

1946–1947: Charles H. Matson—Venice, FL (DDS 1916)

1947–1948: J.F. Spencer[b]—Grand Rapids (DDS 1913)

1948–1949: Laverne H. Andrews—St. Joseph (DDS 1918)

1950–1951: David Seligson—Detroit (DDS 1920)

1951–1952: Harlow L. Shehan—Jackson (DDS 1929)

1952–1953: Glenn R. Brooks—Rochester (DDS 1925)

1954–1955:D.M. Teal—Yale (DDS 1921)

1955–1956 R.W. Walmoth—Auburn Hills (DDS 1923)

1956–1957: Raymond A. Hart—Saginaw (DDS 1929)

1957–1958: Floyd. D. Ostrander—Ann Arbor (DDS 1934, MS Endodontics 1940)

1957–1958: Alfred H. Lowther[b]—Detroit (DDS 1916)

1958–1959: Jack P. Beukema—Grand Rapids (DDS 1925)

1959–1960: Murray A. Leitch—Farmington Hills (DDS 1926)

1961–1962: Frederick A. Henny—Boynton Beach, FL (DDS 1935)

1961–1962: Fred Wertheimer[b]—Farmington (DDS 1949)

1962–1963: J. Robert Short—Spring Hill, FL (DDS 1942)

1963–1964: Edward A. Cheney—East Lansing (DDS 1942, MS Orthodontics 1944)

1964–1965: Kenneth J. Ryan—Flint (DDS 1932)

1967–1968: O. Lee Ricker—Grand Rapids (DDS 1934, MS OMS 1947)

1968–1969: William E. Brown—Ann Arbor (DDS 1945, MS OMS 1947)

1973–1974: Max S. Hart—Flint (DDS 1930)

1974–1975: H. Ward Fountain—Sun City, AZ (DDS 1945)

1975–1976: Joseph M. Cabot—Unknown (DDS 1945, MS Ped Dent 1947)

1976–1977: Richard A. Shick—Flint (DDS 1954, MS Periodontics 1960)

1980–1981: William M. Creason—Grand Haven (DDS 1945)

1981–1982: Robert E. Doerr—Traverse City (DDS 1950, MS Op Dent 1953, Interim Dean 1981–1982)

1983–1984: Wilbert C. Fletke—Lansing (DDS 1945)

1985–1986: Anthony E. Dietz—Bloomfield Hills (MS Endodontics 1955)

1988–1989: David F. Cooley—Kalamazoo (DDS 1966)

1989–1990: Eugene L. Bonofiglo—Grand Rapids (DDS 1958)

1990–1991: John G. Nolen[b]—East Lansing (DDS 1958)

1991–1992: Lawrence R. Marcotte—Grand Rapids (DDS 1967, MS Endodontics 1972)

1992–1993: Ronald J. Paler—Westland (DDS 1961)

1993–1994: Jay A. Werschky—Flint (DDS 1976)

1995–1996: Arnold M. Baker—Holland (DDS 1968, MS Res Dent 1976)

1997–1998: Richard L. Jankowski—Lansing (DDS 1976)

1998–1999: Michael D. Jennings—Grosse Pointe (DDS 1977)

1999–2000: Gary L. Zoutendam—Battle Creek (DDS 1973)

2000–2001: Robert D. Mitus Jr.[b]—Grand Rapids (DDS 1978)

2003–2004: Raymond F. Gist—Flint (DDS 1966)

2004–2005: George T. Goodis—Grosse Pointe (DDS 1964)

2005–2006: Josef N. Kolling—Ann Arbor (DDS 1981, MS Rest Dent 1984)

2007–2008: Steven M. Dater—West Michigan (DDS 1988)

2008–2009: Joanne Dawley—Detroit (DDS 1980)

2009–2010: William L. Wright—Jackson (DDS 1975, MS Ortho 1984)

2011–2012: Connie M. Verhagen—Muskegon (DDS 1986, MS PedDent 1988)

2012–2013: Jeffery W. Johnston—Sterling Heights (DDS 1982, MS Periodontics 1986)

2015–2016: Mark M. Johnston—Lansing (DDS 1985)

2017–2018: Michele Tulak-Gorecki—Warren (DDS 1990)

a  Dentist initially trained under a preceptor before the dental school was established in 1875.

b  Honorary President

# Index